Operative Extraction of Wisdom Teeth

OPERATIVE EXTRACTION OF WISDOM TEETH

Peter Tetsch and Wilfried Wagner

Translated by Claire Shellis and R. P. Shellis

PSG PUBLISHING COMPANY, INC.
LITTLETON, MASSACHUSETTS

Printed by Ebenezer Baylis & Son Ltd, Worcester

Originally published in Germany, under the title
'Die operative Weisheitszahnentfernung' 1982
(Carl Hanser Verlag München Wien)

Distributed in North America and Canada by
PSG Publishing Company, Inc.
by arrangement with Wolfe Medical Publications Ltd

Library of Congress Cataloging in Publication Data

Tetsch, Peter.
Operative extraction of wisdom teeth.

Translation of: Die operative
Weisheitszahnentfernung.
Bibliography: p.
Includes index.
1. Molars—Surgery. 2. Teeth—Extraction.
I. Wagner, Wilfried. II. Title. [DNLM: 1. Molar,
Third—surgery. 2. Tooth Extraction. WU 605 T3470]
RK531.T4813 1985 617.6'6 85-583
ISBN 0-88416-539-6

CONTENTS

FOREWORD

The wisdom teeth, as a result of their particular topography, phylogeny and ontogeny, are directly or indirectly the underlying cause of numerous disorders in the mouth, jaw and facial regions. As a result their removal is often necessary and wisdom tooth extraction is the most frequently undertaken oral surgical operation.

The authors have described in detail the multitude of surgical, orthodontic and prosthetic problems associated with the wisdom teeth, so that the reader is informed not only about the various disorders and illnesses and the most expedient surgical techniques, but also about the indications for removal or conservation of the wisdom teeth. The inclusion of sections on anaesthesia, technical equipment and apparatus required, possible complications and their control and the procedure with high-risk patients has resulted in a comprehensive work which will undoubtedly contribute to the improvement of the treatment of wisdom tooth disorders.

Each section of the book shows the great personal experience of the authors which, backed by a sound understanding of the underlying theory, allows them to describe this extensive area clearly and pragmatically.

Rüdiger Becker

PREFACE

The extraction of wisdom teeth is the most frequently performed surgical operation in dental practice; in West Germany more than 100 000 operations of this sort are carried out each year. However, numerous papers and publications show that this operation is often underestimated and is associated with a multitude of intra- and post-operative complications. This results in the referral of patients to specialist clinics when they have been treated in a general dental practice but the operation could not be completed successfully in the surgery.

The book should be an aid both to the student and to the practising dental surgeon in both the hospital and private practice. In addition to the description of the practical procedure, therefore, special attention is paid to pre-surgical diagnosis and to the possible complications which may arise, particularly in older patients, in patients with pathological changes and in high-risk patients.

We thank Professor R. Becker, director of the Department of Oro-maxillo-facial Surgery of the Westphalian Wilhems-University of Munster, for stimulating criticism and valuable advice and also for kindly writing the foreword.

Our thanks are also due to Dr B. Tetsch for correction and stylistic revision of the manuscript and for numerous constructive suggestions, which have contributed to clarity.

Mrs B. Labouvie kindly undertook the extensive clerical work and M. W. Sailer the preparation of the diagrams.

This book will have fulfilled its aim if it makes a contribution towards the prophylactic, early removal of wisdom teeth and the reduction of the complication rate.

P. Tetsch
W. Wagner

1 INTRODUCTION

'Wisdom teeth ensure the perfection of the whole'
Bergemann (1981)

In Tibetan philosophy, wisdom teeth have a special significance; only upon the appearance of the third molars are the pre-ordained relationships of the individual teeth to one another, the preservation of harmony, the balance and perfection of the whole achieved.

In contrast to this view is the reality of dental practice, in which the wisdom tooth is regarded as just a problem. It can lead to serious disturbances in the harmony of the masticatory apparatus and the general state of health, and is often responsible for a host of complications. It influences the planning and treatment in all dental specialties and forms a focal point in dental surgery.

According to Ricketts (1980) it is believed that about half of the population need to have their third molars removed before the age of thirty. The main cause of the high incidence of this operation lies in the phylogenetic regression of the jaws and the resulting lack of space. The evolution of *Homo sapiens* has been accompanied by a reduction of the jaws which must be related to alteration in dietary conditions and habits. That is to say, functional stimulation must be regarded as one of the primary stimuli for development of the jaws. In this context, the absence of the phenomenon of attrition of the approximal contacts on molars and premolars plays a part. Such attrition has been known since Philips (1931) and Ackerman (1934) and leads to mesial drift of the cheek teeth which, in the case of very rigorous masticatory demands, such as can still be found among primitive peoples, may amount to as much as 10 mm. Here the problem of the crowded wisdom tooth does not exist. Elastic deformation of the jaws, intra-alveolarly damped vibration of the teeth and tooth eruption have been discussed as causes of attrition (Geheb, 1981).

The *regression of the jaws* is connected with a *reduction* in the *number of teeth*. If one compares the general dentition of mammals with that of man, a systematic reduction is seen, in each case of the last teeth in a group, i.e. the lateral incisors, the second premolars and the distal molars. Krekeler *et al.* (1974) established from 1614 patients that in 10.5% all four wisdom teeth, and in 28.2% of cases at least one wisdom tooth, had not formed.

According to Lytle (1980), less than 5% of adults with the full complement of teeth have sufficient room for the complete eruption of the third molars where these develop. Thus the third molars play a predominant role in the incidence of retention.

With retention can be connected infections, cysts, tumours, neuralgiform pain, anomalies of tooth position, masticatory dysfunction, disturbances of occlusion and myoarthropathies.

While as recently as 100 years ago the removal of wisdom teeth was an operation which was carried out very infrequently, and only with severe complications, it is now considered a routine procedure. In the Poliklinik for Dental Surgery at the University of Mainz, it is the most frequently performed operation, comprising 30% of total operations. Nevertheless, it is an operation with a relatively high complication rate, which increases among older patients and occasionally leads to claims for legal liability. The most common complications are disturbances of sensation, residual root tips, infections of sockets and fractures of the jaw. The complication rate can be considerably reduced by early removal of the wisdom teeth.

2 GENERAL PRINCIPLES

Wisdom tooth rudiments show up on radiographs between the seventh and tenth years of life. Mineralisation of the crown of the tooth can first occur at this age. The time when eruption occurs varies considerably; it is quoted as around the twentieth year on average.

Before eruption of the tooth, the inner and outer enamel epithelia, which are in contact following the regression of the stellate reticulum, are adjacent to the crown of the tooth. The epithelium first becomes detached from the outer enamel surface after fusing with the oral epithelium (**1**). This pericoronal space is

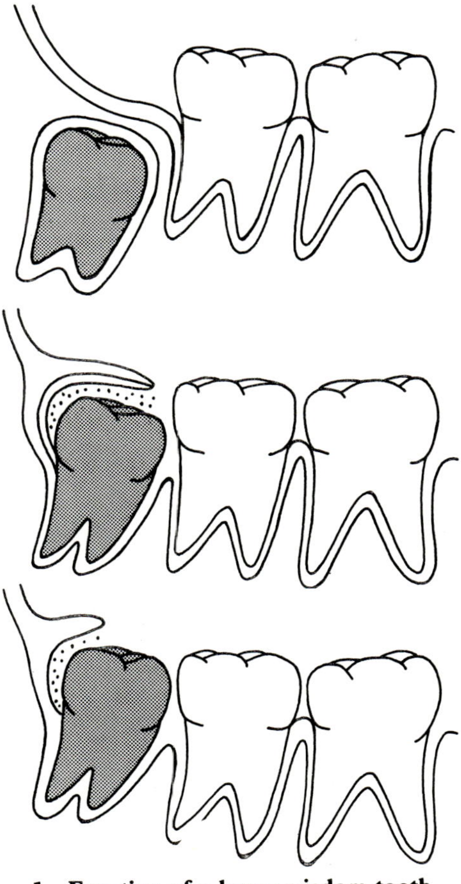

1 Eruption of a lower wisdom tooth.

bordered on the inside by enamel and on the outside by the dental follicle together with the enamel epithelium. It forms an ideal trap for bacteria, food residues and cell debris, which opens up with continuing eruption of the tooth and disappears completely in the normal course of events. A trouble-free eruption is only possible, however, if the crown of the tooth contacts gingiva which is firmly bound to the periosteum. In lower wisdom teeth especially, often only the mesial cusps can erupt, due to lack of space, while the distal cusps impinge on the mobile alveolar mucosa. This is merely raised up and continues to lie over the crown. Since the eruption of the tooth proceeds not at all or only very slowly beyond this stage, the distal pericoronal space remains as a permanent food trap (see Section 3.2.1).

Wisdom teeth show a great degree of variation in the proportion of root and crown. Recurved root tips, which can seriously complicate surgical procedure, often occur (**111, 112**). Occasionally, rudimentary tooth germs are also observed (**2**).

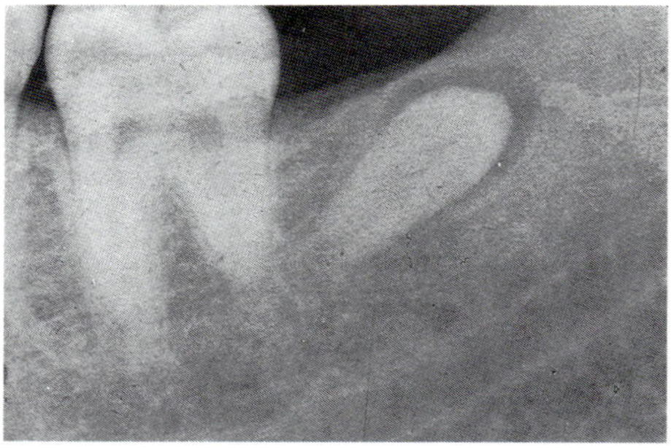

2 **Rudimentary wisdom tooth in left mandible.**

With advancing age, an involution of the periodontium sets in. It involves reduction of periodontal cell activity, a narrowing of the periodontal space, a thickening of the cortical bone and a reduction of the spongiosa. Numerous complications of surgical procedure are connected with this.

2.1 Definitions (Table 1)

When a tooth, following completion of root growth, fails to reach the occlusal plane, one refers to this as *retention*. If the tooth remains within the jaw and is surrounded by bone, it is a case of *complete retention.* Distinguished from this are teeth which perforate the mucosa with only part of the crown. In this case we have *partial retention*, or half retention. If a tooth is prevented from erupting by adjacent hard structures (teeth, tumours) or is embedded in bone on all sides, this is referred to as *impaction*. This is therefore a form of retention. The concepts of impaction and retention are indeed applied synonymously. If the axis of the tooth is rotated through 180°, this is referred to as *inversion*.

A further classification of types of retention is set out in Section 2.4.

A *displacement* (dystopia dentium) exists if the teeth do not occupy their usual place in the dental arch. After only partially erupting, they remain fixed, orientated either along the direction of eruption or irregularly. The term displacement is also used synonymously with retention or impaction.

In extreme cases, 'stray' teeth occur (heterotopy, aberratio dentium). These can result from dispersal or, rarely, from migration of the tooth bud, in the embryo.

Table 1 Retention (failure to reach the level of the occlusal plane)

Total (complete) retention, Surrounded by tissue on all sides
Partial retention (half retention), Perforation of the oral mucosa by the crown

2.2 Causes of retention

Many possible causes of retention have been discussed. In individual cases, a cause is often difficult or impossible to identify. Lack of space is undoubtedly of prime importance if there is a discrepancy between the number or size of the teeth and the size of the jaw (**3**). This disparity can be determined relatively simply. According to Ricketts (1980), this is already possible at 9 to 11 years of age and even earlier. A prediction of the size and shape of the lower jaw can be made with an accuracy of 95% by means of cephalometric investigations. The growth of the ascending ramus and of the articular process proceeds primarily in the cranial and dorsal directions, while the anterior border of

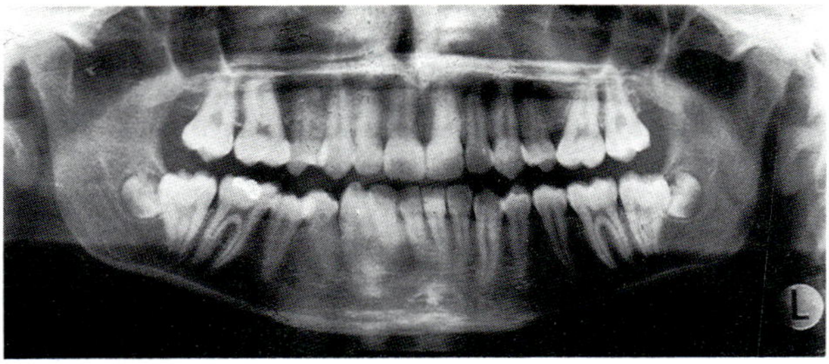

3 Orthopantogram of a 12-year-old youth. Mineralised crowns of the lower wisdom teeth. Agenesis of the upper wisdom teeth. Extreme lack of space.

the mandible changes only slightly (**4**). If the distance from the centre of the ascending ramus to the distal border of the second molar amounts to 30 mm in a fully grown person, the prognosis for normal eruption is very good. The critical value is around 25 mm.

The cause of the lack of space lies in the phylogenetic regression of the jaw, which is connected with a reduction of the dentition. Enlargement of the brain case is accompanied by a reduction in size of the facial skeleton. A disparity between the sum of the widths of the teeth and the size of the jaw results. The wisdom teeth, which develop last, therefore have insufficient space for correct eruption.

Along with these measurable factors, there are a large number of other possible causes which are relatively easy to recognise if they are considered as mechanical hindrances of eruption,

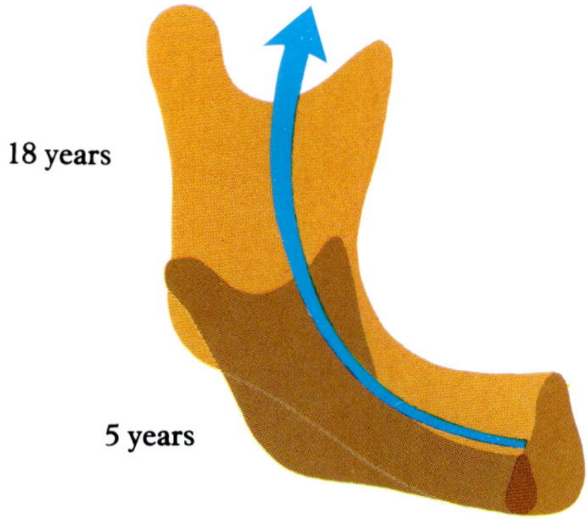

4 Growth curve of the mandible (modified from Ricketts, 1980).

namely pathological changes such as fusion of teeth (**5**), cysts (**6**), tumours (**7**), tissue hyperplasias or localised infections. In

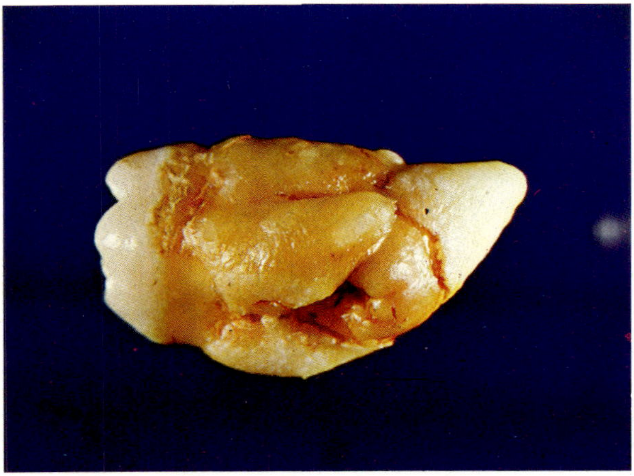

5 Fusion of an upper wisdom tooth with the second molar. Interradicular position of the tooth crown.

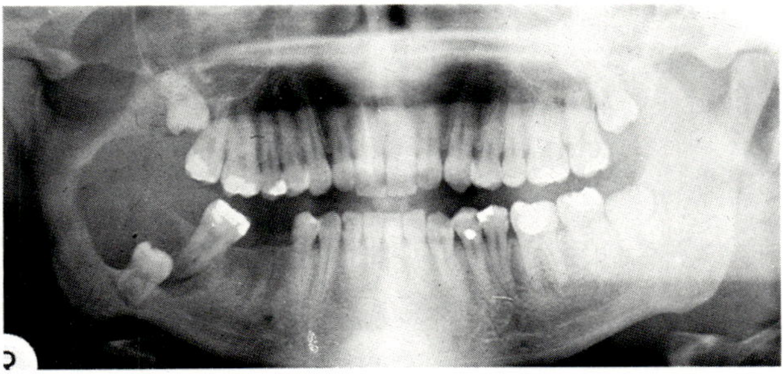

6 Follicular cyst of the right ascending ramus with retention of lower right wisdom tooth.

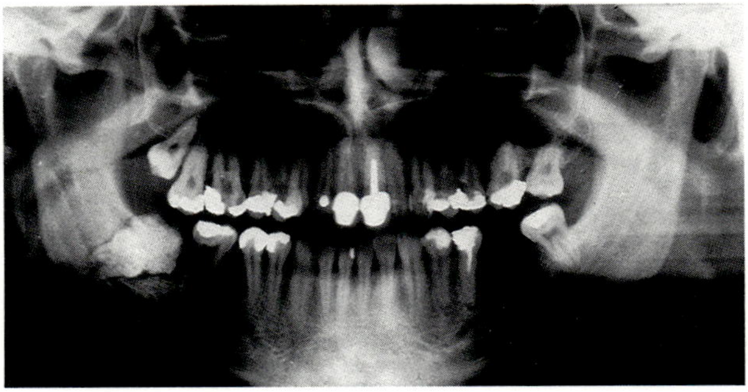

7 Complex odontome as an obstruction to the eruption of impacted lower right wisdom tooth.

addition, traumatic and hereditary influences, vitamin A and D deficiency and endocrine factors can be regarded as potential reasons for retention. Impressive multiple tooth retention can be observed in specific syndromes (e.g. cleidocranial dysostosis; **8, 9**) or other generalised conditions (e.g. congenital hydrocephalus, cretinism, mucopolysaccharidoses; **10**: Spranger, 1978).

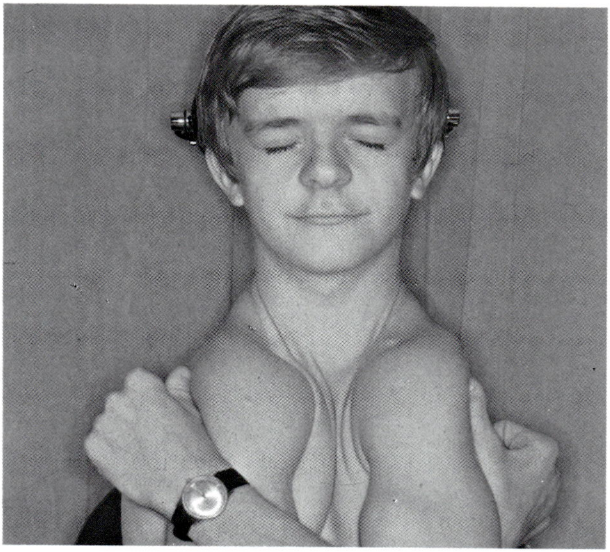

8 Aplasia of both clavicles in cleidocranial dysostosis in a 15-year-old patient.

If there is no apparent cause for a hindrance of eruption, a lack of eruptive force is frequently to blame. In our own biometric studies it could be ascertained that, although in a high percentage of cases there was lack of space, retention without obvious clinical grounds was also seen not infrequently.

2.3 Frequency of retention

The wisdom teeth are – due to their late development – by far the most frequently retained teeth. In a study of 3874 patients by Dachi and Howell (1961), it was established that after their twentieth year, 17% of the patients had at least one retained tooth. Mead (1930) reported on 581 retained teeth, of which 461

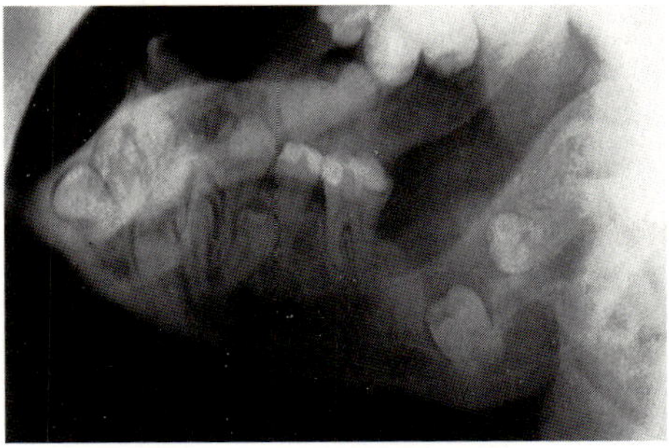

9 Multiple retentions and supernumerary teeth in cleidocranial dysostosis (see **8**).

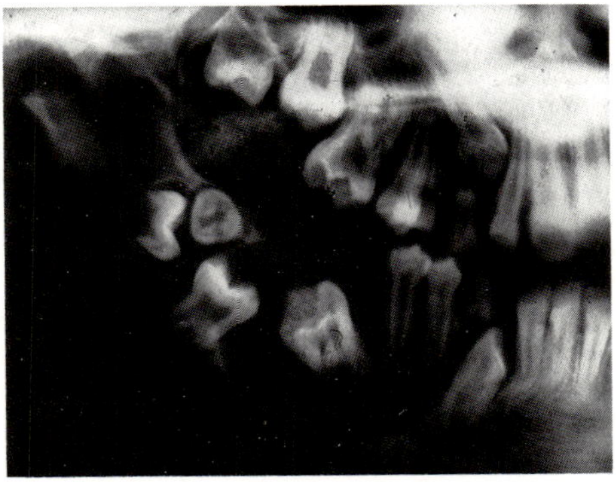

10 Multiple retention, distomolars, cystic changes, hypoplastic alveolar processes in a case of Type VI mucopolysaccharidosis.

(79.3%) were wisdom teeth. According to information from the West German Federal Dental Association (Kassenzahnärztliche Bundesvereinigung) for 1980, 179 057 retained and displaced teeth were removed by osteotomy from national health patients in West Germany. This included, along with wisdom teeth, canines, premolars, supernumerary rudimentary teeth and other teeth. In our own practice, a statistical evaluation of 1000 such osteotomies gave the following proportions expressed as percentages:

Wisdom teeth	78.0%
Canines	13.9%
Premolars	4.6%
Supernumeraries	3.1%
Others	0.3%

If one assumes a similar percentage distribution, it follows that in West Germany, over 140 000 displaced and retained wisdom teeth are removed surgically each year.

2.4 Types of retention

The type of retention has a decisive influence on the surgical procedure and determines to a large extent the degree of difficulty of the operation. A classification is therefore appropriate:

- vertical retention – approximately parallel with the adjacent molars, ca. 90° to the occlusal plane,
- horizontal retention – approximately parallel with the occlusal plane, ca. 0°,
- inclined retention – sloping at a large variety of angles to the occlusal plane,
- aberrant retention.

Within the types of retention listed above, further divisions are possible (Table 2).

Table 2 Summary of types of retention

1.	Vertical retention		
2.	Horizontal retention		
	2.1	Sagittal	
		2.1.1	Mesioangular
		2.1.2	Distoangular
	2.2	Transverse	
		2.2.1	Buccoangular
		2.2.2	Linguo-angular
3.	Inclined retention		
	3.1	Mesioangular	
	3.2	Distoangular	
	3.3	Buccoangular	
	3.4	Linguo-angular	
4.	Aberration		

2.4.1 Vertical retention

The types of retention can also be expressed by an angular measurement in a circular diagram. The long axis of the wisdom tooth is related to a line drawn above the cusps of the molars and premolars on an orthopantomogram. If the angle between the two lines approaches 90°, it is a vertical retention. The crown of the tooth points towards the occlusal plane. When 1000 patients were evaluated, all the wisdom teeth whose axes formed angles of 80–100° with the reference plane were defined as vertically retained (**11–14**).

The vertical type of retention occurs in the lower jaw in 38.2% and in the upper jaw in 62.9% of cases.

2.4.2 Horizontal retention

A horizontal retention exists if the angle described lies between 350° and 10° or between 170° and 190° (**11, 12** and **15, 16**).

At the angles specified, only sagitally orientated, horizontally retained teeth are recognised. In addition, displacement in the transverse direction is possible (**17, 18**).

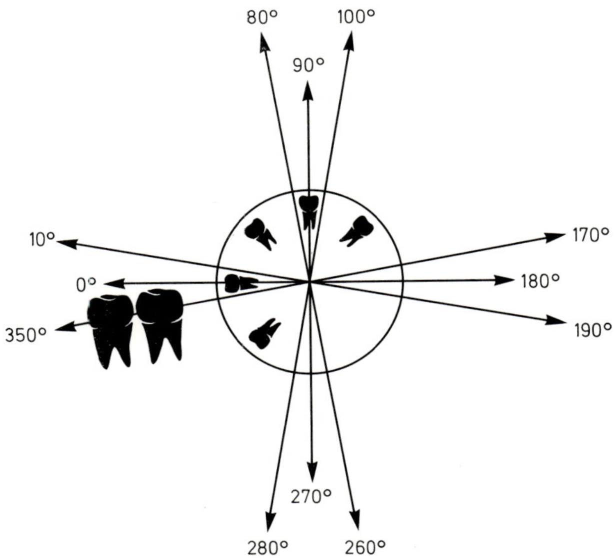

11 Diagram showing the angles for the possible types of retained wisdom teeth in the left mandible.

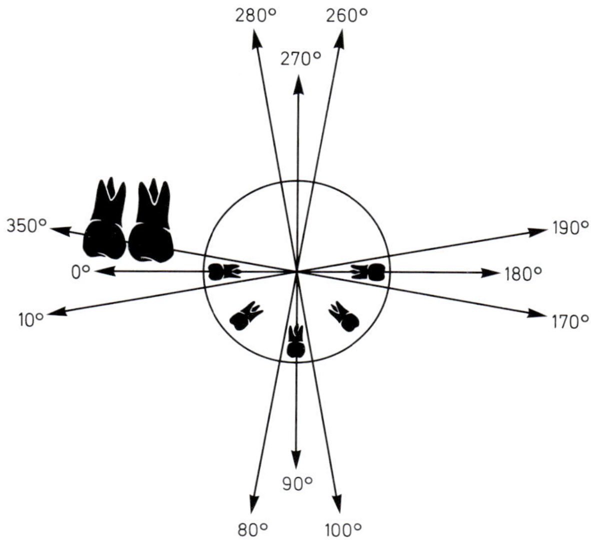

12 Diagram of the angles for the possible types of retained wisdom teeth in the left upper jaw.

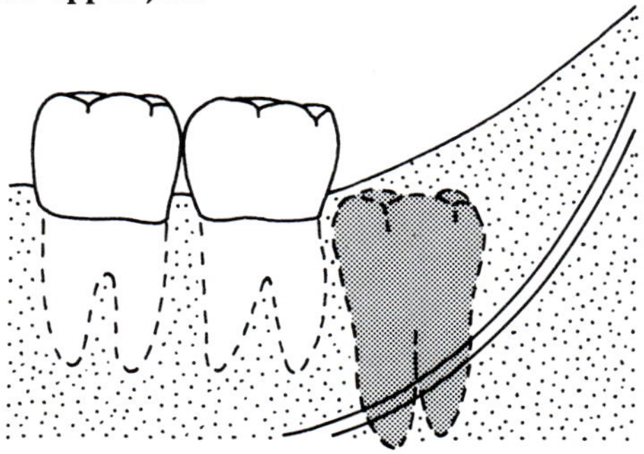

13 Diagram of a vertically retained lower wisdom tooth.

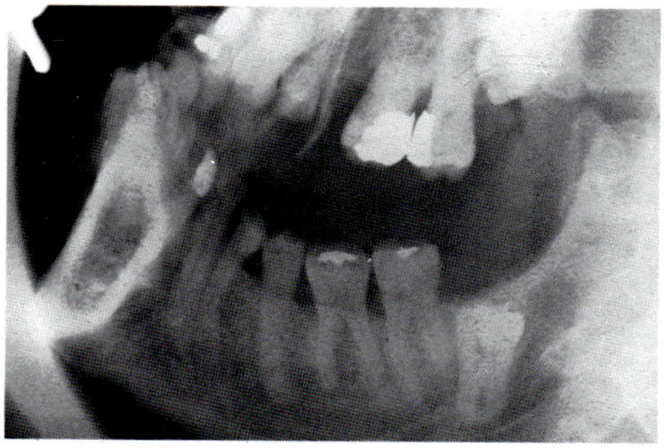

14 Radiograph of a vertically retained lower wisdom tooth.

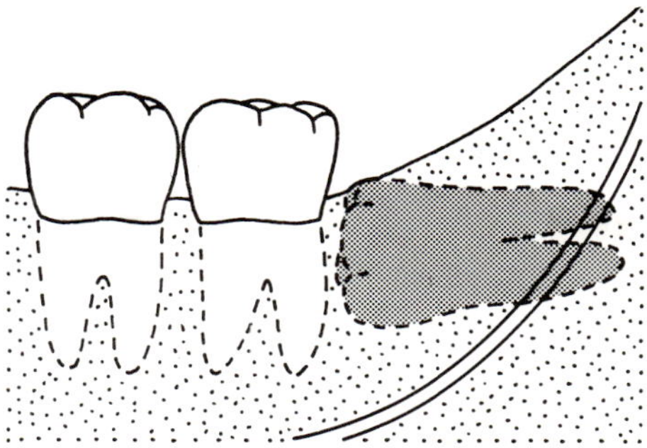

15 Diagram of a horizontally retained lower wisdom tooth in the mesioangular position.

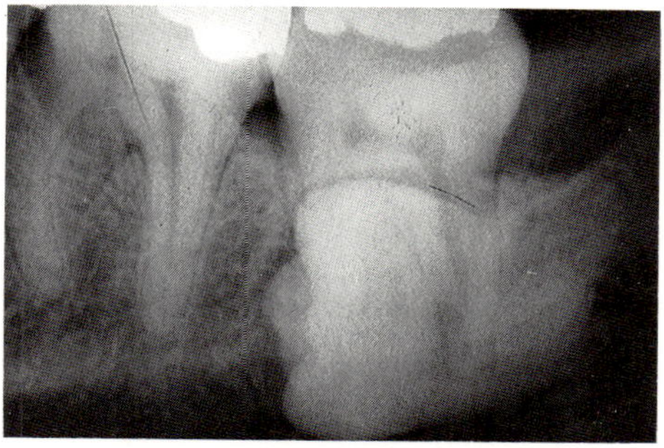

16 Radiograph of a horizontally retained lower wisdom tooth in the mesioangular position.

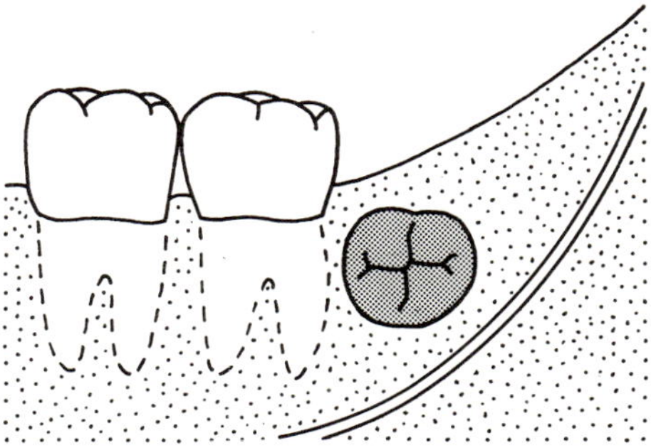

17 Diagram of a retained, transversely displaced lower wisdom tooth.

The frequency of horizontal retentions is 11.2% in the lower jaw and 0.1% in the upper jaw. No distoangular positions have been found in the lower jaw and no mesioangular positions in the upper. Horizontal transverse retentions are very rare (upper jaw 0.3%, lower jaw 1.3%).

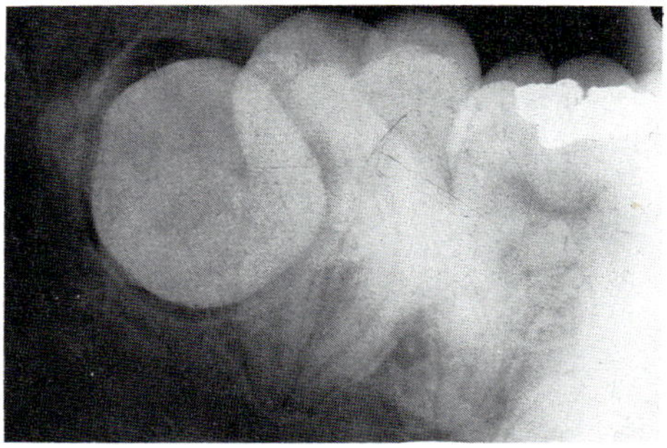

18 Radiograph of a transversely retained lower wisdom tooth (buccoangular).

2.4.3 Inclined retention

All teeth which lie between the angles mentioned above are referred to as inclined. According to the position of the crown, they are divided into mesio- or distoangularly inclined types of retention (**19–22**).

While in the lower jaw inclined mesioangular retention is the most common, with an incidence of 43.6%, in the upper jaw distoangularly inclined types of retention are predominantly observed (24.6%). The percentage distribution, using the same circular diagram, is shown in **23, 24**.

In the lower jaw 93% of the teeth are orientated between 350° and 100° (**23**); in the upper jaw 99% lie between 10° and 170° (**24**).

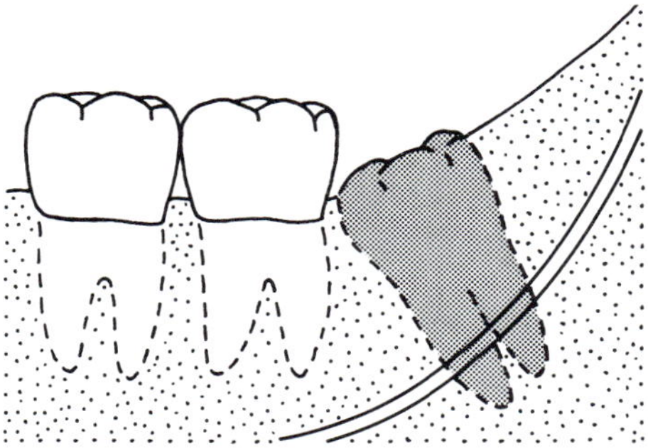

19 Diagram of inclined retention (mesioangular) of a lower wisdom tooth.

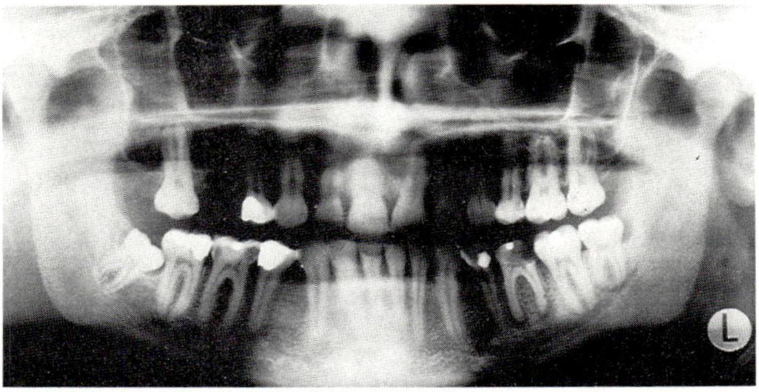

20 Radiograph of an inclined right lower wisdom tooth in the mesioangular position.

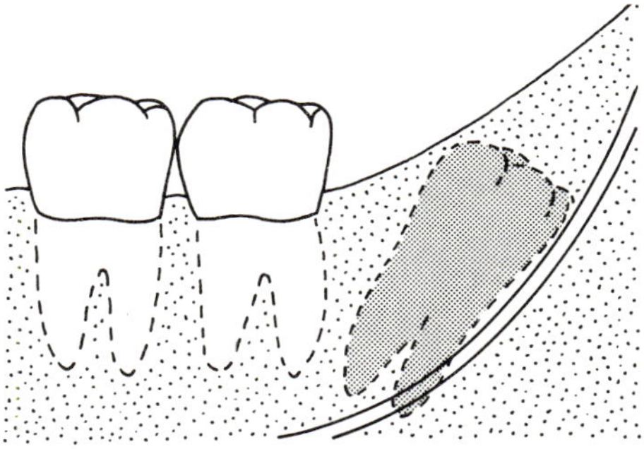

21 Diagram of inclined retention (distoangular) of a lower wisdom tooth.

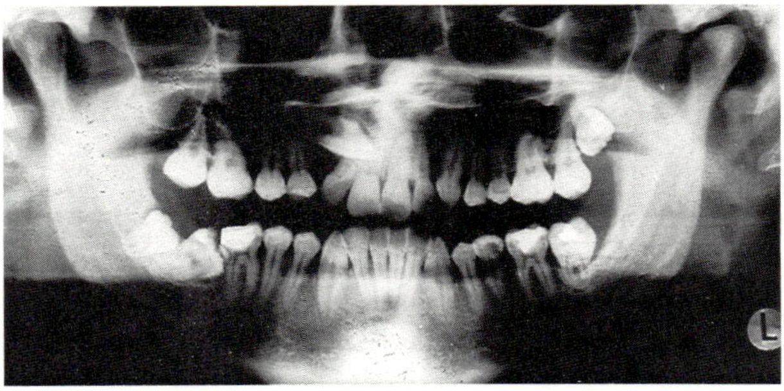

22 Radiograph of an inclined retained upper left wisdom tooth in the distoangular position. Lower right second and third molars in the mesioangular inclined position.

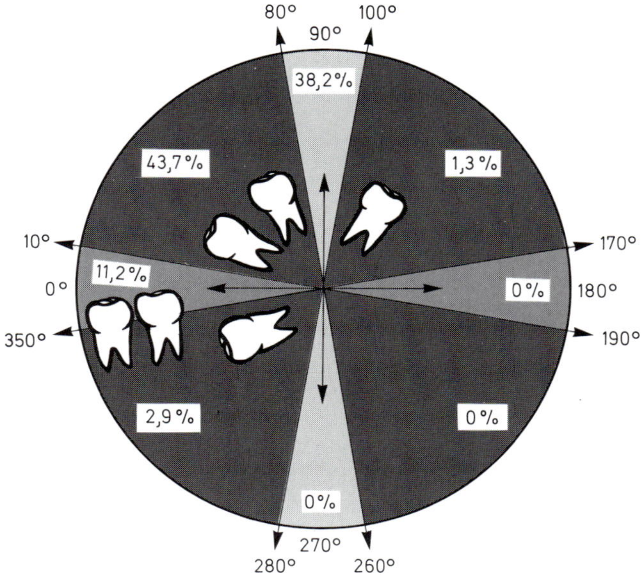

23 Percentage distribution of the types of retention of the lower wisdom teeth from an evaluation of 1000 orthopantograms.

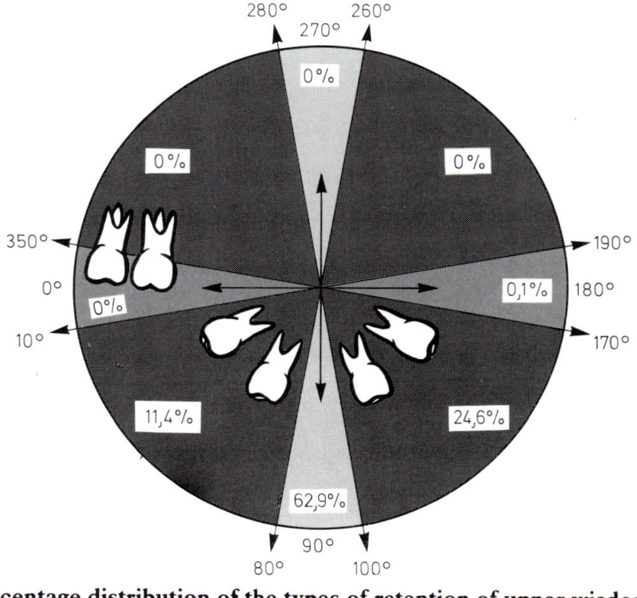

24 Percentage distribution of the types of retention of upper wisdom teeth.

In contrast to these retentions in the sagittal plane, retentions in the transverse plane can also occur. Depending on the direction of the crown of the tooth, the retention is either linguo- or buccoangular.

2.4.4 Aberration

Occasionally, aberrations are observed. In the upper jaw, the aberrant teeth are predominantly found in the vicinity of the maxillary sinus (**25**), while lower wisdom teeth may be located in the ascending ramus (**26**) or at the base of the mandible (**27**). Aberrations are more common in the upper jaw (1.3%) than in the lower (0.7%).

Equally rare are inverted teeth, which we have not observed in our studies.

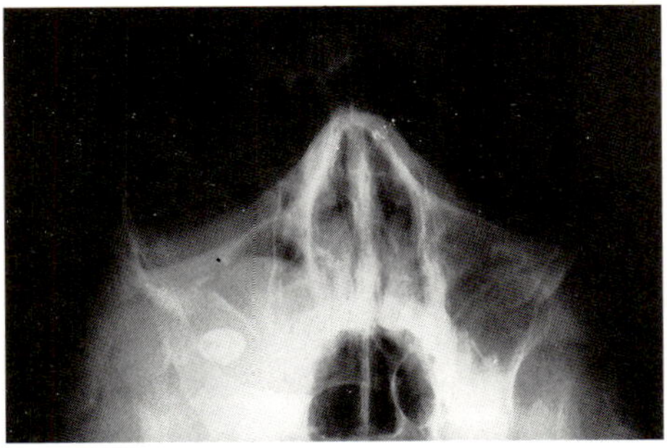

25 Aberrant upper wisdom tooth in the right maxillary sinus (**nasal cavity radiograph) with extensive follicular cyst.**

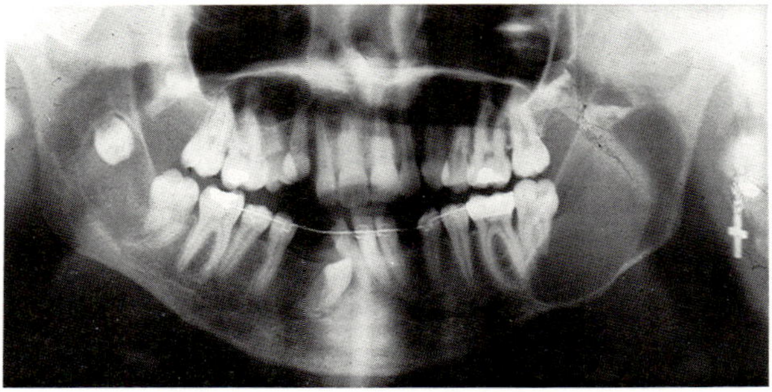

26 Aberrant lower wisdom teeth in connection with follicular cysts; on the left the mineralised crown of the wisdom tooth can be seen in the muscle process of the right ascending ramus.

2.5 Assessment of the situation

In the case of partially retained wisdom teeth a clinical examination gives immediate information about the type of retention. Nevertheless, a radiograph before the surgical operation is imperative. The radiograph will give information about:

- the type of retention,
- the condition of the crown and roots,
- the relationship of lower wisdom teeth to the inferior dental canal (only possible in the vertical type) and to the adjacent teeth,
- type and extent of pathological changes (tumours, cysts, fractures).

These requirements are met by *survey radiographs* (orthopantomograms, lateral radiographs of the body of the mandible or of the ascending ramus and lateral Status-X radiographs). Intra-oral films are often insufficient to clarify the situation and will only suffice in favourable cases, since the extent of pathological changes and their relationship to neighbouring structures often cannot be assessed. The intra-oral film is so positioned between jaw and tongue that the film surface and the axis of the tooth are parallel. In the case of small films (3 × 4 cm), the front edge of the film should coincide with the mesial edge of the first molar, or better still bisect the first molar. The upper edge of the film must lie in the same plane as the occlusal surface of the first and second molars. With size 4 × 5 cm films the front edge of the film should coincide with the mesial edge of the second premolar.

While, as a rule, radiographs in one plane will suffice, in some circumstances radiographs in *two dimensions* are necessary to assess the situation. This is so for horizontal, transversely displaced teeth, for large cysts and all malignancies and for fractures.

A Clementschitsch radiograph can show the lateral extent of pathological processes, dislocations in the case of fractures of the angle of the jaw and the state of the crown in the case of transversely displaced teeth (**28**).

Donovan (1952) and others have described *axial projection methods* in which the intra-oral film lies against the anterior edge of the ascending ramus with the mouth either in the biting position or wide open. The central ray passes from the outer angle of the jaw perpendicularly on to the film. However, these radiographic techniques have not proved useful (Becker, 1961). The parallax technique, using two intra-oral radiographs in each case, gives better information on the position of the tooth. One radiograph is set up in the orthoradial position and another in the mesio- or disto-eccentric position (**28, 29**). A further parallax investigation can also be carried out, in which apart from the orthoradial radiograph another one is shot at an angle of −15° to −25°. Since with the displacement of the central ray, objects

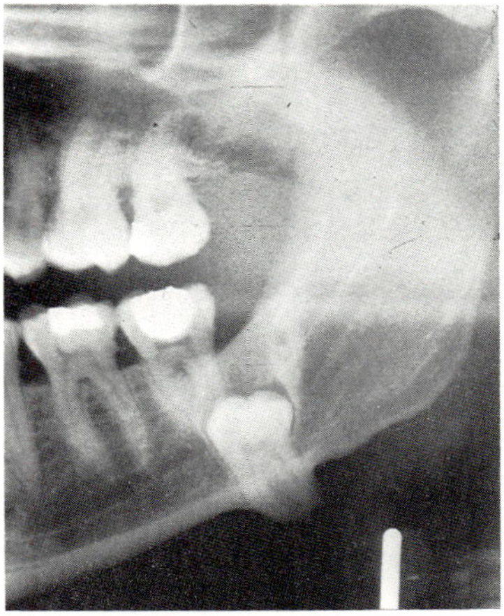

27 Aberrant wisdom tooth at the base of the mandible.

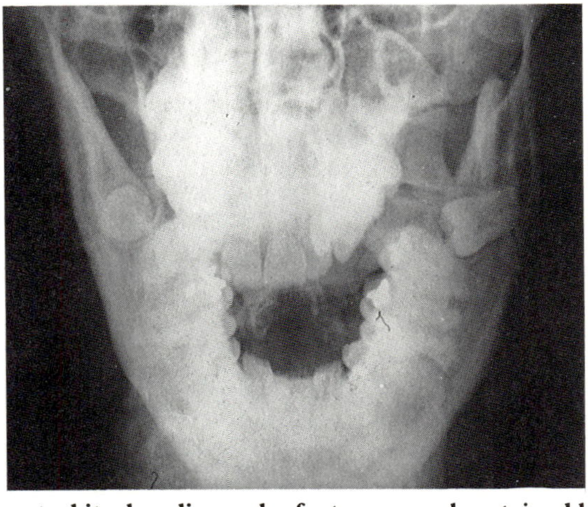

28 Clementschitsch radiograph of a transversely retained lower right wisdom tooth, linguo-angular position.

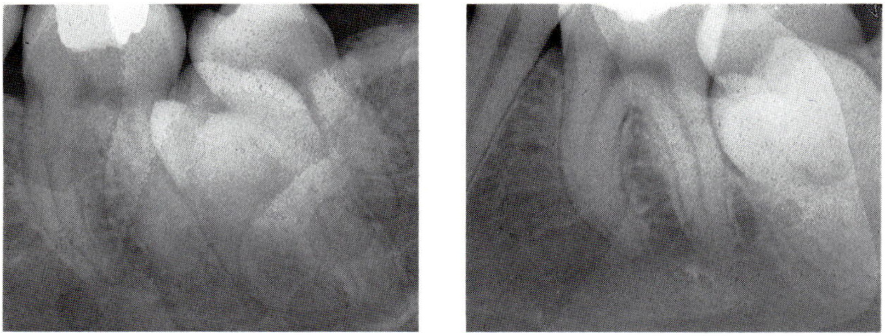

29 Parallax investigation to establish the crown position of a transversely displaced lower wisdom tooth. Left: orthoradial; right: mesio-eccentric. The wisdom tooth is lying further away on the eccentric plate and shows a greater displacement than the second molar. It therefore lies further away from the film (= vestibular).

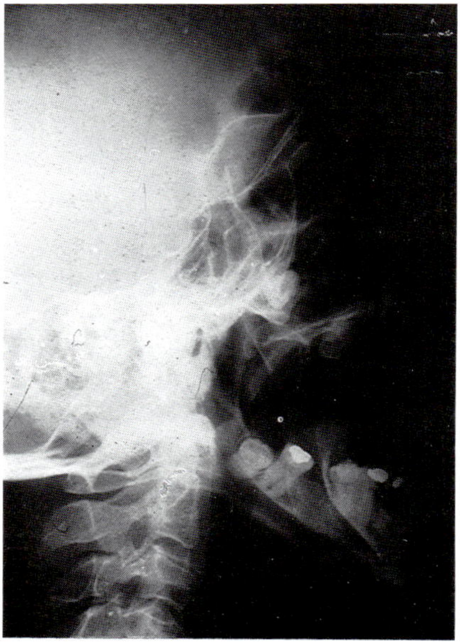

30 Lateral cranial radiograph to locate an aberrant upper wisdom tooth.

close to the film shift less than those further away, and in addition give a less sharp contrast, an idea of the orientation of the individual parts of the tooth and of its relationship to the neighbouring teeth can be gained. However, parallax procedures are of only minor clinical importance in wisdom tooth diagnosis and are only rarely necessary for ascertaining the type of retention.

In the upper jaw a nasal cavity radiograph should be taken if cysts or malignancies are suspected or when there are dystopic teeth. In the case of drastically displaced or aberrant wisdom teeth a lateral cranial radiograph may also be necessary (**30**).

2.6 Age of the patient, timing of the operation

Age of the patient

Varying opinions are held concerning the most favourable time for surgical extraction of wisdom teeth. They range from extreme restraint, when an operation is only considered at the onset of severe complications, to the prophylactic removal of the unmineralised tooth germs at the age of 9 years. By means of cephalometric studies it is already possible at this age, according to Ricketts (1980), to make an accurate prediction of the growth of the mandible and the expected availability of space. The accuracy of these long range predictions is quoted as 95%. On the basis of these studies, the early removal of wisdom teeth is recommended in the American literature. According to Ricketts (1980), even the germs of the third molars in the lower jaw should be removed between 9 and 11 years of age when there is the threat of impaction.

However, operations on children are not without problems. This is especially true for the upper jaw, where the tooth in an 8–10-year-old child may lie very high, its removal is difficult and traumatic, and the possibility of damage to the second molars cannot be excluded. Therefore, to us the 12–18 year age group – after the eruption of the second molars at the earliest – seems more suitable. Here, moreover, a decision about the eventual situation can be arrived at by analysis of a survey radiograph without expensive cephalometric investigations.

If there is extensive crowding, removal of teeth should be carried out at this age. Early extraction has the following *advantages*:

Surgery relatively straightforward because of

- wide pericoronal space,
- incomplete root development,
- straight roots,

- infrequent contact with the inferior dental canal,
- infrequent contact with the maxillary sinus,
- no pre-operative infections,
- reduced danger of fracture,
- good general health.

Surgery has possible *disadvantages*, which become more significant with advancing age.
Operation is complicated by

- completed root development,
- enlargement of the teeth,
- curved roots,
- calcification of the root surface,
- frequent contact with the inferior dental canal,
- frequent contact with the maxillary sinus,
- pre-operative infections,
- general illnesses.

This comparison shows that early removal is preferable. However, until now it has played a subordinate role. The differentiation of 1335 patients by age shows that in less than one-third of cases (27.1%) was the operation carried out in the second decade of life (**31**). The maximum (42.8%) lies in the

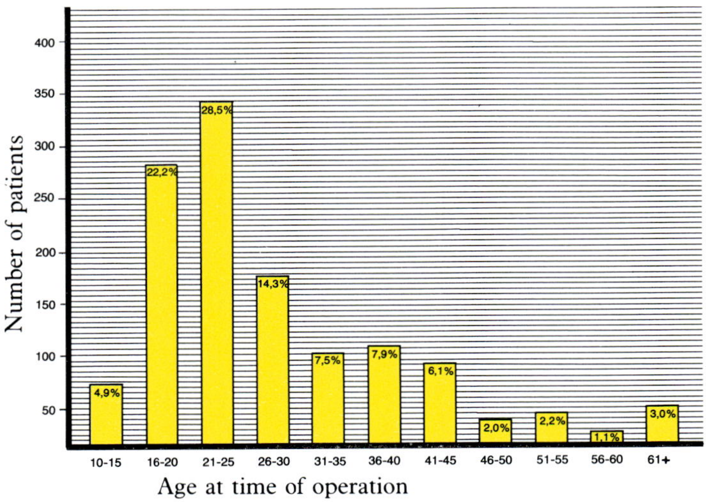

31 Frequency distribution according to age at time of operation (analysis of 1335 patients).

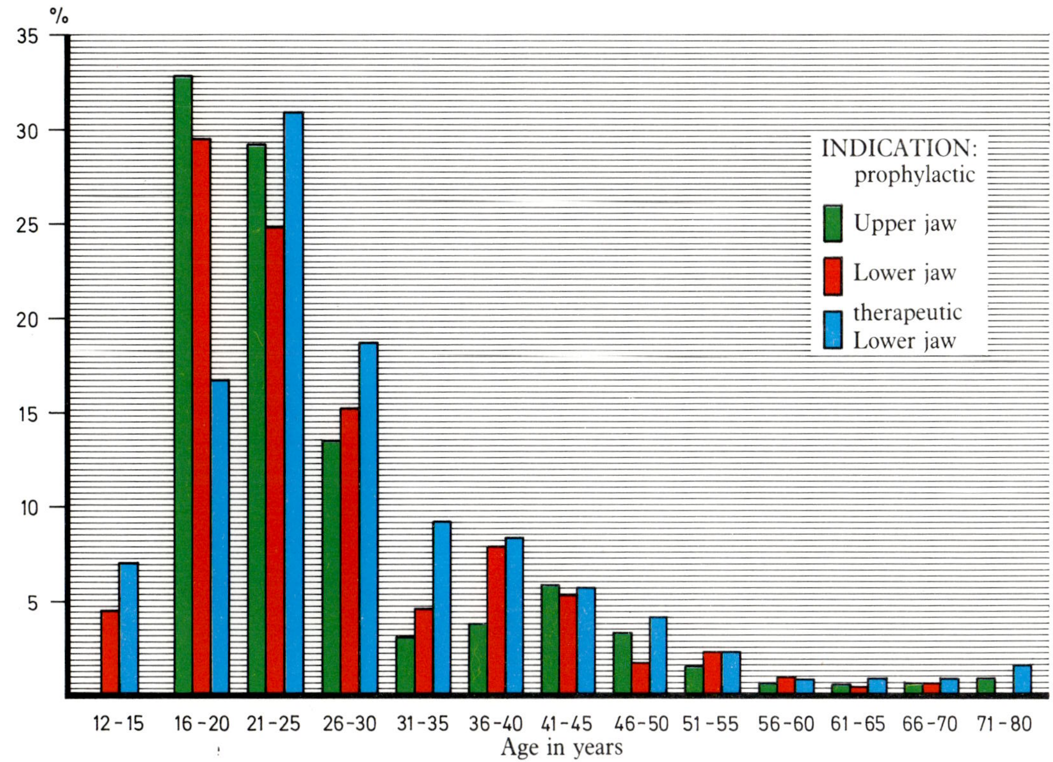

32 Frequency distribution of the age at operation in relation to the indication (analysis of 1000 patients).

third decade of life. In the majority of cases in this age group, inflammatory complications are the reason for the extraction. Subdivision into prophylactic and therapeutic indications shows a significant shift in the age maxima (**32**). In the 12–15 year age group, wisdom tooth germs are removed exclusively prophylactically for orthodontic reasons. This indication also predominates on a per cent basis in the 16–20 age group, although therapeutic cases are also seen here. The latter have their maximum between 21 and 25 years and predominate until 35 years of age. Wisdom teeth also continue to cause problems in the higher age groups. Even in the over-60 age group, wisdom teeth were removed from 40 patients (0.3%).

Timing (day of the week)

Deciding on the most favourable day of the week depends on the particular organisation of the practice. Since experience has shown us that swelling and subjective pain are greatest on the second and third post-operative days, an inspection of the wound should take place, or at least be possible, on the second day. Any necessary drainage of the wound should also be removed or changed at this point in time (see Section 4.6). As a rule, a certificate of inability to work will also be required for this period. It is particularly difficult to decide on the timing if the patient is going on holiday in the near future. If less than ten days are available, it is often better to confine oneself to the treatment for a pericoronitis and postpone the extraction until the return of the patient.

Above all, in the case of complicated impactions, sufficient time should be allowed for surgery to enable one to operate at leisure.

Even the choice of the *time of day* can be important. It should be early in the morning in the case of diabetics and patients with a tendency to haemorrhage in order, with the former, to take advantage of the optimum metabolic state and with the latter to have a long period for observation and after-care.

3 INDICATIONS FOR SURGICAL REMOVAL

Wisdom teeth should always be removed if they are diseased and cannot be preserved. Their removal is likewise indicated if deleterious effects are encountered or are expected in their vicinity and if they are completely non-functional and may become merely a source of complications. In assessing the indications, both the local condition of the whole masticatory system (extended local condition) and the general condition of the patient should be taken into account.

A large number of contra-indications prohibit a surgical procedure. Extraction should be avoided if the stress of the operation and the damage it would cause outweigh the condition which would result, and the complications which would be expected, from leaving the wisdom tooth in place.

In this connection, local factors and generalised illnesses play a role. In old age, particularly, problems occur owing to a general lowering of the state of health and to atrophied jaws. The risk of spontaneous fracture and damage to nerves as a result of surgery increases in proportion to advancing age. The operation itself is more difficult and after-care more prolonged.

In young patients, surgery can be contra-indicated by haemophilia, leukaemia or the after-effects of radiotherapy.

On the basis of the contra-indications described, especially among older patients, early extraction of the wisdom teeth seems prudent.

Surgical extraction of wisdom teeth is regarded as a routine operation these days. An increasing trend towards prophylaxis as a favourable indication can be observed. The reasons for this lie in the development of modern local anaesthetics, which render the operation completely pain-free, and in improved surgical techniques. Antibiotics, general social security and an increasing receptivity towards prophylactic measures all play a further part in this development.

The analysis of 500 patients, from whom a total of about 1000 wisdom teeth were removed surgically, shows a predominance of prophylaxis as an indication (Table 3).

Since inflammatory complications only occur rarely in the upper jaw and since we favour the simultaneous extraction of both wisdom teeth on one side under local anaesthesia, the therapeutic indication plays only a subordinate role here.

Table 3 Indications for extraction of wisdom teeth

	Upper jaw (%)	Lower jaw (%)
Prophylactic indication	89.2	62.2
Therapeutic indication	10.8	37.8

3.1 Prophylactic indications

3.1.1 Lack of function

Retained wisdom teeth can perform no masticatory function. They are therefore just a possible source of complications and should be extracted if normal eruption is not expected and no further treatment possibilities are indicated. The latter could consist of orthodontic adjustment, extraction of molars or a transplant.

Orthodontic adjustment of a retained wisdom tooth into its correct position continues to be restricted to extremely rare and exceptional situations. It is a different matter if prematurely decayed molars have to be extracted. According to Baume (1940) the systematic extraction of the first molars should be carried out if at least three molars are decayed.

Schwarz (1942) advises that one should also extract first permanent molars which are not expected to be conservable until the third decade of life. The most favourable time to extract them is at 10–11 years of age, since at this age the wisdom teeth are easier to visualise radiographically, as described in Section 2.2, and the second molars have erupted. In these cases, there is a high probability that the gap will close completely due to the pressure of growth of the wisdom tooth. The longer extraction is delayed, the greater is the danger of the second molar tilting forwards. Expensive orthodontic measures with fixed appliances are then necessary to restore the correct position.

The extraction of extensively decayed and unsalvageable second molars can bring about the adjustment of a wisdom tooth. This is possible if the position in the jaw is suitable and the development of the roots not completed. On the other hand, extraction of a healthy second molar to improve the position of the wisdom tooth is to be condemned.

A description of the orthodontic possibilities and procedures is not within the scope of this work. It can be found in the orthodontic literature.

In certain circumstances the experiment of transplanting a wisdom tooth into a molar socket may be carried out. The problems of this procedure are described in Section 5.6.

3.1.2 Infection prophylaxis

The eruption of the wisdom teeth generally proceeds very slowly on account of the weak eruptive force. According to Wassmund (1935) the lower wisdom tooth in particular has to overcome considerably more resistance than the other teeth. The distal portion of its crown is often hindered by the ascending ramus; a strong and firm layer of bone must be broken down. The mucous membrane covering the alveolar process is especially thick and firm on the inner angle of the jaw. These anatomical characteristics encourage the appearance of the symptoms which are collectively known as pericoronitis. They are due either to a persistence of the mucous membrane over the crown or to an infection of the dental follicle (see Section 3.2).

Only rarely does one succeed in avoiding these difficulties by removal of the mucosal flap which is completely or partially covering the tooth, since as a rule there remains a distal bony pocket, which is not in practice amenable to therapy.

The situation is additionally complicated by the fact that there is frequently a zone where attached gingiva is not present in the vicinity of the angle of the jaw. Pockets resulting from tension on the alveolar mucosa can likewise lead to infection. The second molar can also become involved if a deep pocket forms in the bone between it and the wisdom tooth. The whole area is inaccessible to hygienic measures, so the extraction of the wisdom tooth serves as a mode of infection prophylaxis.

Special attention must be paid to patients who are undergoing radiation or immunosuppressant therapy. If the jaw region lies in the field of the radiation, it is considerably damaged by the ionising rays. A radio-osteomyelitis can result from inflammatory complications, often necessitating extensive jaw resection. It should be remembered that all irradiations of the head and neck regions are significant and if in doubt in these cases, one must ascertain whether the jaw lies in the radiation field.

Partly retained wisdom teeth should where possible be extracted before therapy of this sort, since if an operation

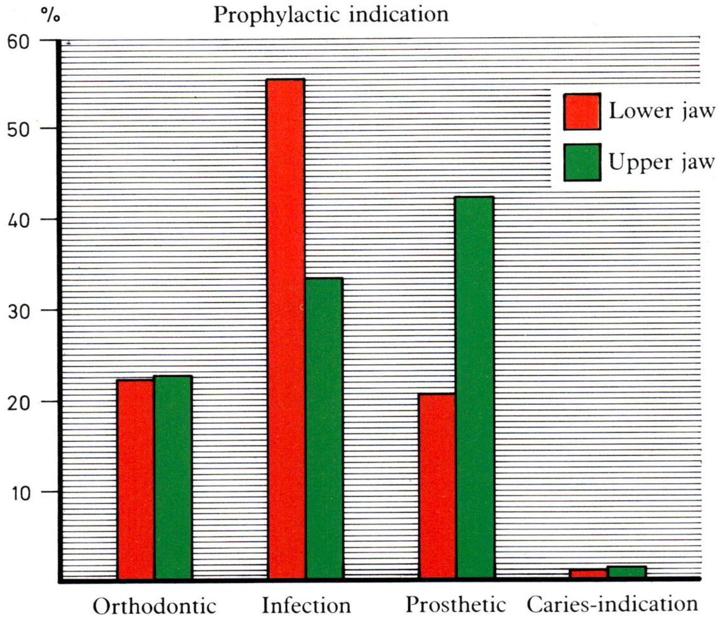

33 Percentage distribution of prophylactic indications for wisdom tooth extraction (analysis of 1000 patients).

becomes necessary later it may be accompanied by great difficulties and – with sufficiently urgent indications – can only be carried out while taking precautionary measures.

Among the prophylactic indications, infection prophylaxis has the greatest significance. 55.9% of lower and 33.3% of upper wisdom teeth are extracted on these grounds in our practice (**33**).

3.1.3 Orthodontic prophylaxis

Many observations suggest that the pressure of erupting, crowded wisdom teeth causes a mesial pressure on the teeth anterior to them and can bring about tertiary overcrowding. Schwarze (1973) has demonstrated the influence of the wisdom teeth on the anterior tooth region by means of comparative studies. Anterior crowding may, it is true, have other causes as well, since it is also observed in cases where the wisdom teeth have not developed or have been extracted. This mesial pressure may represent a threat to the success of orthodontic treatment. The prophylactic extraction of wisdom teeth on orthodontic

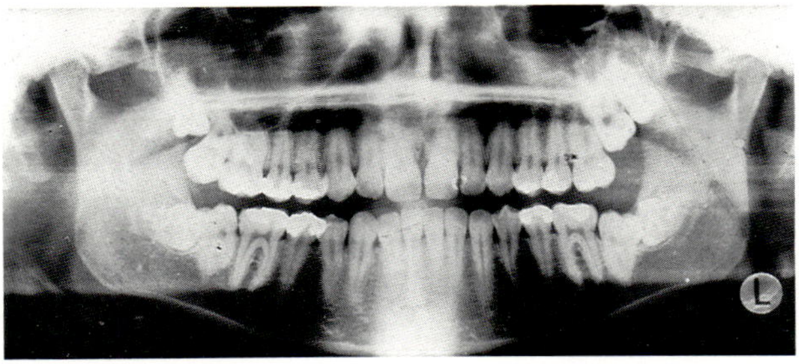

34 Orthopantogram of a 19-year-old patient. Impacted wisdom tooth, partly impacted second molar. Horizontally displaced lower wisdom teeth are hindering the eruption of the respective second molars.

grounds was already advocated by Andresen (1935); however removal of tooth germs has not generally become widespread. Results of treatment by this operation have only recently been published. Pape and Ikemura (1979) report on prophylactic removal of tooth germs in 525 children. The orthodontic indication is based on four conditions:

- lack of space,
- therapeutic borderline cases, instead of extraction of the premolars,

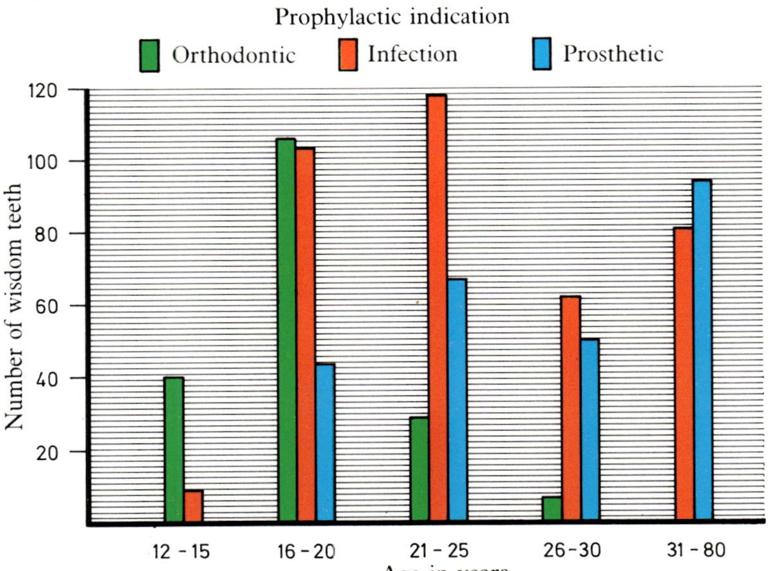

35 Number of wisdom teeth extracted surgically for prophylactic reasons in different age groups.

- distal movement of the premolars and molars with extra-oral appliances,
- completion of orthodontic treatment with first signs of renewed crowding of the incisors.

The preferred age was 14–16 years. Removal of tooth germs should halt the pressure in the mesial direction which is continuous during the period when the child is growing. Kühr and Wetzstein (1970) observed facilitated gap closure when the wisdom teeth were established and improved chances of distalising the cheek teeth if they had not developed or had been extracted. They found an acceleration of the eruption of the third molars following the extraction of posterior teeth, which was greater the further distally the latter were located and the earlier they were extracted. Agenesis of premolars affects the wisdom teeth only by reduction of support and by the mesial movement of the first molar which this involves. In rare cases, wisdom teeth can also hinder the eruption of the second molars (**34**). In an evaluation of 500 patients, 22.6% of the upper and 22.5% of the lower wisdom teeth were extracted in the course of orthodontic treatment. Preventing relapse of completed orthodontic treatment played a major role in these cases (**33**).

While most prophylactic extractions on orthodontic grounds are carried out under the age of 20 years, in the 20–30 year age group infection prophylaxis increases (**35**).

As would be expected, prosthetic indications play a greater role in old age.

3.1.4 Prosthetic indications

Retained wisdom teeth should be removed before crowning the second molars; otherwise they may endanger the prosthetic work by the pressure of growth. Moreover, the periodontal condition changes following osteotomy and may necessitate renewal of crown or bridge work.

Retained teeth can also lead to problems in the case of dentures borne on the gingivae. With increasing atrophy of the alveolar crest, an 'eruption', which may lead to considerable difficulties for denture wearers (**36**) is still possible. This is also true for local inflammatory complications and general illnesses, which at this age can be relative or absolute contra-indications for a surgical operation. Therefore, retained wisdom teeth should be removed before making dentures to be carried by the gingivae.

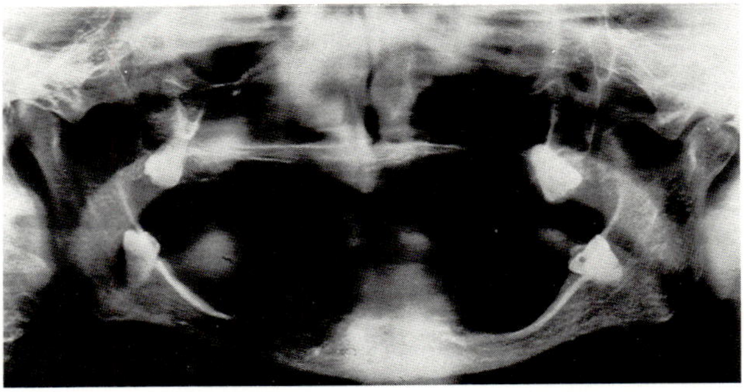

36 Retained wisdom teeth in an 80-year-old patient, which have perforated the mucous membrane and have made the wearing of dentures impossible.

In addition, wisdom teeth can influence the occlusion in various ways. Retention can lead to over-eruption of the antagonist and hence to disturbance of the occlusal equilibrium. Motsch (1977) has reported on this complication, which is also possibly due to the mesial pressure of the wisdom teeth. As a result of a traumatised occlusion, there may arise temporomandibular-joint disorders which, in favourable cases, may be successfully treated by tooth extraction alone.

3.1.5 Oral surgical indications

Wisdom teeth *in a fracture line* must be removed, since they can lead, especially in the case of partial retention, to infection in the fracture (**37**). Fractures in tooth-bearing regions of the jaw are

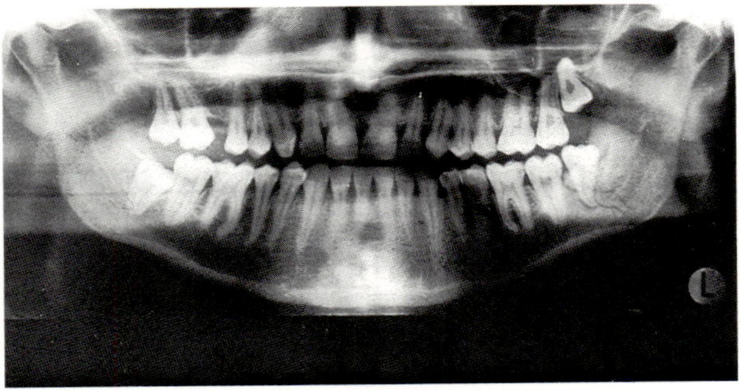

37 Fracture in the angle of the left mandible. Lower left wisdom tooth in the fracture line.

designated open fractures, since through the periodontium a connection exists between oral cavity and bone. The danger of infection is therefore always present. Osteomyelitis was observed in 39 cases out of 860 fractures of the mandible (4.4%; Tetsch *et al.*, 1972). The most common site was the angle of the jaw.

A further indication, from the point of view of oral surgery, belongs to the province of *orthopaedic surgery*. Of special importance is prognathism. The lower wisdom teeth lie in the osteotomy region and can lead to inflammatory complications just as in the case of fractures; they also result in a reduced surface area for bone deposition. Moreover, the pressure they exert can lead to an increased risk of relapse following backward displacement of the mandible.

3.1.6 Damage to neighbouring teeth

Especially in the case of inclined wisdom teeth in the mesioangular position, damage to the second molars may occur. Thus, carious defects or resorptions are often found in the region of contact (**38**). Possible damage to the tooth supporting tissues has already been referred to (**39**).

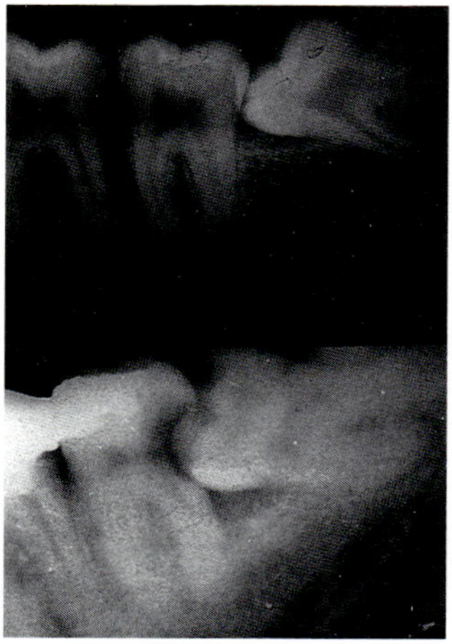

38 Inclined lower left wisdom tooth in contact with second molar (above). 15 months later, considerable damage to the crown of the second molar (below).

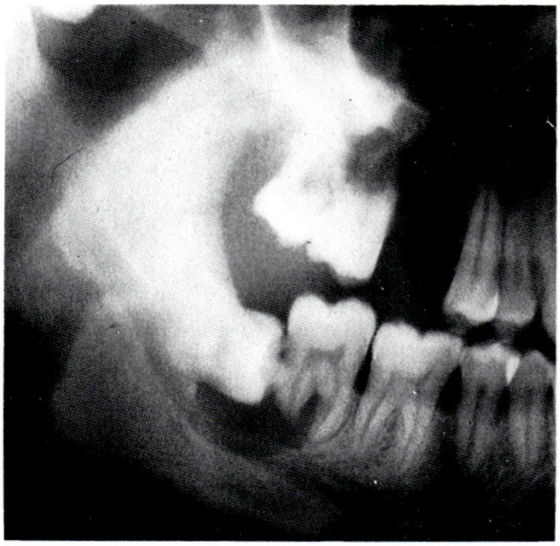

39 Follicular cyst on lower right wisdom tooth with resorption of the distal root of the adjacent second molar. Extensive destruction of tooth support.

3.2 Therapeutic indications

3.2.1 Pericoronitis

Pericoronitis is generally understood as a complication of wisdom tooth eruption, especially in the lower jaw, which is usually accompanied by inflammatory processes of varying severity. The term therefore comes to be applied synonymously to these

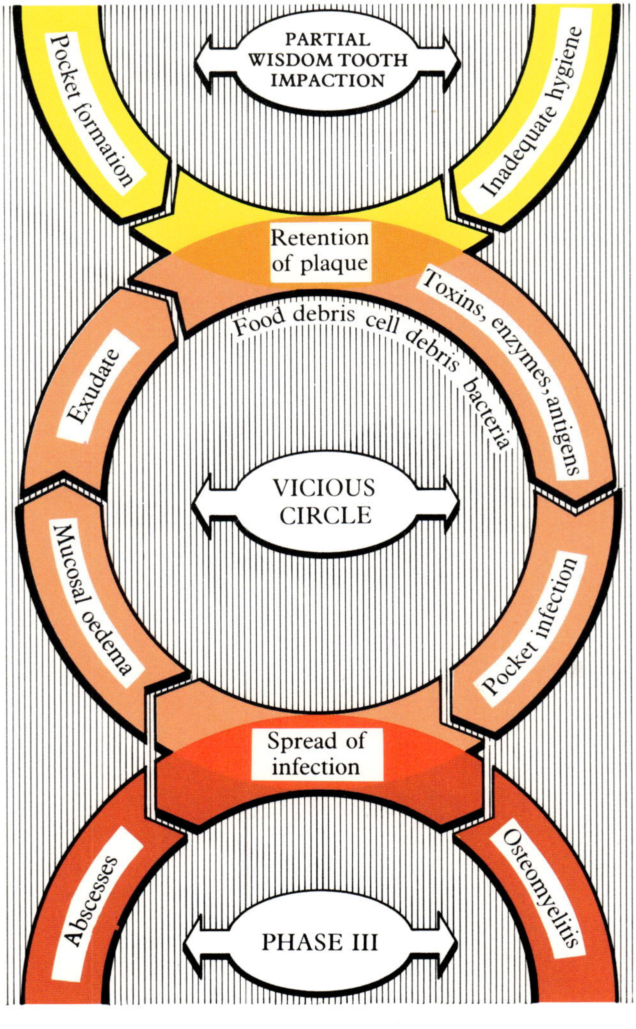

40 The vicious circle in pericoronitis.

inflammatory processes. Pericoronitis is the third most common of the odontogenic infections, with an incidence of 6.5%, after periapical periodontitis (68%) and alveolitis (25%) (Schmelzle and Schwenzer, 1981). Wessels (1978) found the following figures among patients at the Clinic for Maxillo-facial Surgery at the University of Mainz: periapical periodontitis 47%, alveolitis 31%, pericoronitis 10%. In our practice, pericoronitis is the main causative factor in therapeutic extraction of lower wisdom teeth (72.9%) and is often the first indication to both patient and dentist of a retained wisdom tooth.

Pathogenesis and symptomatology

The pericoronal pocket offers, with its uniform, partly anaerobic, incubator-like conditions, the ideal environment for infection of debris in a soft tissue crevice. This leads, as does occasional occlusal trauma, to oedematous swelling of the gingivae and hence to a vicious circle where the symptoms are maintained because the drainage of secretions has been hindered (**40**).

Pericoronitis of the wisdom tooth is thus primarily an inflammatory complication of eruption, which occurs in the surrounding mucosa. Intra-orally, local swelling, reddening and sensitivity to pressure are observed in the region of the pocket (**42, 43**). A purulent discharge is exuded either spontaneously or under pressure from the pericoronal space. As a result of accompanying osteitis, a distinct bony pocket often forms distally, which augments the infection (**41**). As a rule, the pulp is healthy; only occasionally do deep carious defects in cases of long-standing partial retention result in inflammation of the pulp, i.e. necrosis with periapical periodontitis, and with their complications simulate a pericoronitis in the form of inflammation of the soft tissue at the site of eruption (**44**).

Depending on the virulence of the bacteria, the degree of resistance and local conditions, the *oedema* begins to *spread* through the action of toxins. This is accompanied by local swelling, reddening and pain. If there is further oedema, it leads very rapidly to separation of the lateral pterygoid and masseter muscles, which results in stiffness of the jaw. The onset of difficulty in swallowing indicates spreading into the sublingual space and the anterior palate.

There follows an accompanying lymphangitis or lymphadenitis and a deterioration of the general condition. In most cases a

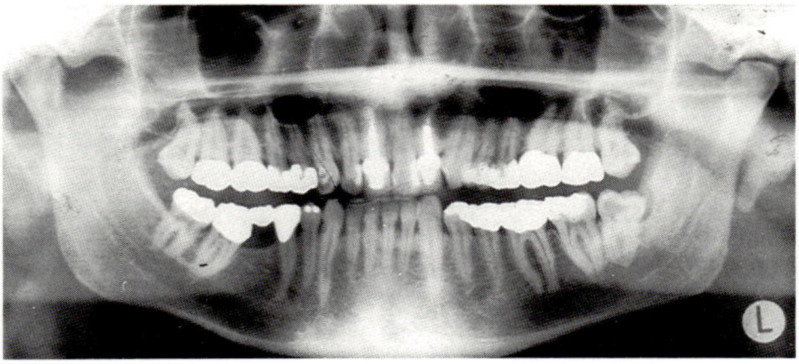

41 Distal infra-bony pocket and carious lesion of vertically retained lower left wisdom tooth.

doughy extra-oral swelling of the region of the angle of the jaw can be clearly seen.

With the spread of infection, *general symptoms* also become evident. These are tachycardia, fever and general malaise, which can be demonstrated by a significant leucocytosis with left shift and by an increased BMR. Within the swelling which spreads to the neck and the tissue of the floor of the mouth, foci of infection and abscess formation may occur, which may then act as a source of infection for the adjacent areas (**45, 46**). Next, perimandibular, pterygomandibular or submasseteric abscesses may spread over the para-pharyngeal space to the mediastinum (mediastinitis) and to the base of the skull (meningitis) and lead to possibly fatal complications. However, this occurs very rarely these days owing to treatment with antibiotics. An evaluation of 3591 clinically treated cases of odontogenic inflammation in the jaw and face region by Schuchardt *et al.* (1964) showed that in a high percentage of cases, space abscesses were a result of pericoronitis (Table 4).

Inflammatory complications occur only rarely in the case of eruption of the upper wisdom teeth, but need special attention on account of the tendency for infection to spread into the infratemporal space. Also in cases of jaw stiffness, decubital

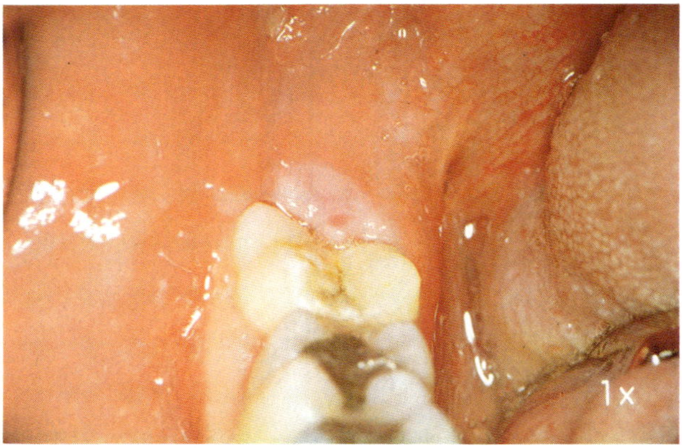

42 Pericoronitis of a partially impacted lower right wisdom tooth with oedematous swelling of the mucosal flap lying on the occlusal surface (Phase I).

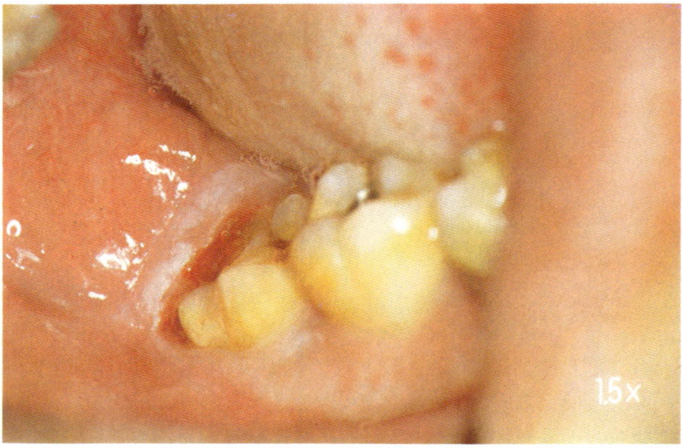

43 Pericoronitis of a partially impacted lower right wisdom tooth with purulent discharge from the distal mucosal pocket. Oedema of the surrounding area (Phase II).

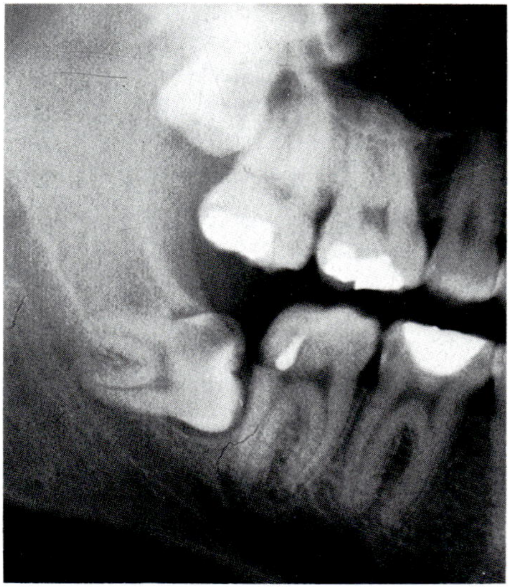

44 Carious lesion in horizontally displaced lower right wisdom tooth (clinically without perforation of the mucosa).

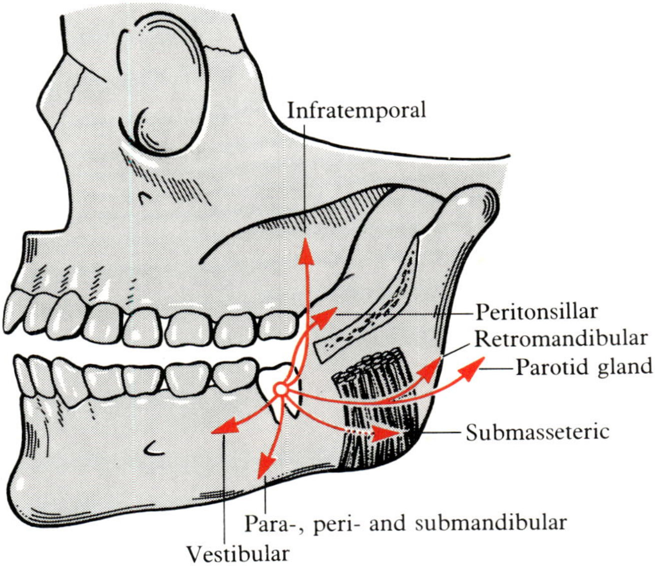

45 Possible spread of inflammation in the region of a pericoronitis of the lower wisdom tooth (from the vestibular aspect).

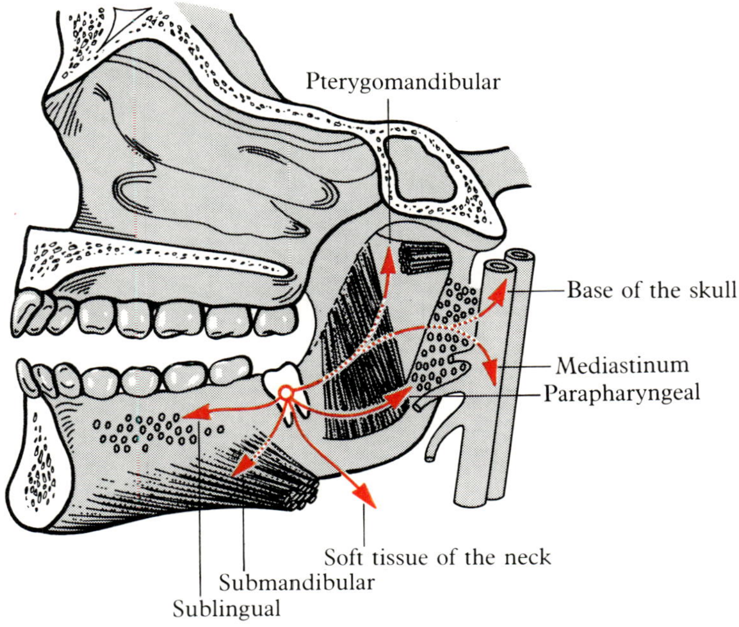

46 Possible spread of inflammation in the region of a pericoronitis of the lower wisdom tooth (from the lingual aspect).

ulcers of the cheek mucosa and local reddening in the first instance, in combination with para- or retro-tubal pain on pressure and especially bilateral oedema of the temples, immediate admission into a specialist clinic is recommended.

Table 4 Wisdom teeth as the cause of odontogenic infections (after Schuchardt *et al.*, 1964)

Location	Lower jaw (%)	Upper jaw (%)
Para-pharyngeal	65.4	—
Pterygomandibular	62.5	—
Paratonsillar	43.5	10.0
Submasseteric	37.0	—
Paramandibular	33.3	—
Perimandibular	27.2	—
Submandibular	22.2	—
Cheek	22.2	—
Sublingual	9.0	—
Infratemporal	—	64.3
Temple	—	15.0

Therapy

The symptoms of *acute exacerbation* and the corresponding therapy can, according to the recommendation of Harnisch (1947), be divided into three phases, between which smooth transitions are possible (Table 5). The basis of a rational therapy is formed by the elimination of the pericoronal pocket by extraction, i.e. surgical removal, of the retained wisdom tooth, which generally has no functional value. A simple removal of the mucous membrane flap leads only in very rare cases to healing, as there is a high incidence of relapse, since a permanent and reliable elimination of the pocket is seldom possible. The reason for this is the distal bony pocket, which is not in practice accessible to therapy. In the phase of local acute exacerbation of the inflammation, it is necessary next to remove the acute symptoms and pain by means of local cleaning, drainage and, eventually, disinfection so that the extraction of the tooth may follow as quickly as possible. In this case we recommend flushing with hydrogen peroxide–Rivanol solution followed by application of a CHKM (chlorophenol–camphor–menthol) gauze strip which is changed daily. We do not consider local application of cortisone-containing ointments or even antibiotic preparations

Pathogenesis	Phase	Clinical signs	Therapy
Partial Wisdom Tooth Retention ↓ **Pocket Formation** Occlusal trauma → Infected gingivae → Influenza-type infections → Food retention → **Soft Tissue Infection** ← ↓ Oedema of flap ↓ Obstruction of flow of secretions ↓	I	Local pain Reddening of the flap Swelling of the flap	Tooth extraction Osteotomy Possible short-term measures as in Phase III
Oedema of Surrounding Tissues (Masticatory musculature, cheeks, gingivae) ↓ **Lymphadenitis**	II	Jaw stiffness Doughy infiltration of the cheek Onset of difficulty in swallowing Pain caused by pressure Swelling of lymph nodes Subfebrile temperature	Cleansing of pocket Disinfection of pocket Drainage of pocket } e.g. flushing with H_2O_2, CHKM gauze strips Antibiotics if infection is spreading; e.g. marked generalised symptoms
↓ **Abscess Formation** ↓ **Spread of Infection** (Focal abscesses, osteomyelitis)	III	Fever Deterioration of general health Marked jaw stiffness Great difficulty in swallowing Severe infiltration	Lancing of abscess Drainage Antibiotics in case of tendency for sepsis to spread

Table 6 Review of antibiotics (selected)

			Example of preparation	Average daily dose
beta-lactam antibiotics	Penicillin (orally active)	Phenoxy-methyl-penicillin	Arcasin Mio Beromycin Mega Isocillin Mega	4 × 1 capsules or 3 × 2 capsules
		Propicillin	Baycillin Mega	
	Cephalosporin (orally active)	Cephradin	Sefril 0.5	4 × 2 capsules
		Cephradoxide	Bidocef	3 × 1 capsules
Macrolides	Erythromycin	Erythromycin	Erythrocin 500	2 × 1 capsules
	Lincomycin	Lincomycin	Albiotic	3–4 × 1 capsules
			Cillimycin	3–4 × 1 capsules
	Clindamycin	Clindamycin	Sobelin	3–4 × 2 capsules
	Spiramycin	Spiramycin	Selectomycin	4 × 2 capsules
Broad-spectrum antibiotics	Penicillin-combinations	Ampicillin + Oxacillin	Totocillin 0.5	4 × 3 capsules
	Tetracycline	Doxycyclin	Vibramycin	1st day 2 capsules then 1 capsule daily

to be advisable. At the onset of a tendency towards spread of infection, with doughy infiltration of the surrounding soft tissue and lymphadenitis together with increasing jaw stiffness and difficulty in swallowing, additional antibiotic therapy and anti-inflammatory treatment may be required, in order to limit the progress of the inflammation. The most common streptococcal/staphylococcal mixed infection can be treated with beta-lactam antibiotics, especially 4 × 1 million International Units or 3 × 2 million IU of an orally active penicillin (Table 6). Apart from allergies, at these dosages no toxic side-effects are to be expected, so that penicillin is the antibiotic of choice. The modern, orally active cephalosporins present an alternative; only in the case of known allergies can antibiotics of the macrolide group be alternatively employed. Broad spectrum antibiotics or combinations with penicillinase-resistant penicillin should be reserved for vital indications in the case of spread of infection, or utilised following an antibiogram in the case of resistant organisms. One must make sure not only of a sufficiently high dose but also, in the case of the frequently short-term acute problems of pericoronitis, of a sufficiently lengthy treatment (three days after end of fever, but at least 8–10 days altogether) in order to avoid the development of resistance. Further details such as side-effects of antibiotic therapy, can be found in appropriate reference sources (Walter and Heilmeyer, 1975).

On transition to the last phase, with abscess formation and marked jaw stiffness, it is necessary to refer the patient to a specialised clinic (**47**). Where the case takes a relatively mild course, with formation of a submucosal abscess along the oblique line with a high point frequently in the region of the first molar, incision of the abscess under local anaesthesia may provide sufficient therapy. Where there is extensive spread of infection, incision and drainage under general anaesthetic is necessary since, first, in most cases extra-oral incision is necessary and, secondly, extensive local anaesthesia is hardly possible because of the stiffness of the jaws in cases where there is acute inflammation in the retromolar space with infiltration of the musculature; and in addition local anaesthesia is contra-indicated on account of the danger of transferring the infection into the pterygomandibular space. The careful management and the extra-oral nerve stem anaesthesia needed to overcome jaw stiffness are seldom applied in this practice and shall only be referred to here, without going into technical details. After the resolution of the acute inflammatory complications, the retained tooth responsible for them may be extracted, usually under local anaesthesia.

Pericoronitis of upper wisdom teeth occurs in only 1% of surgical patients. In the lower jaw, 20% have to receive pre-

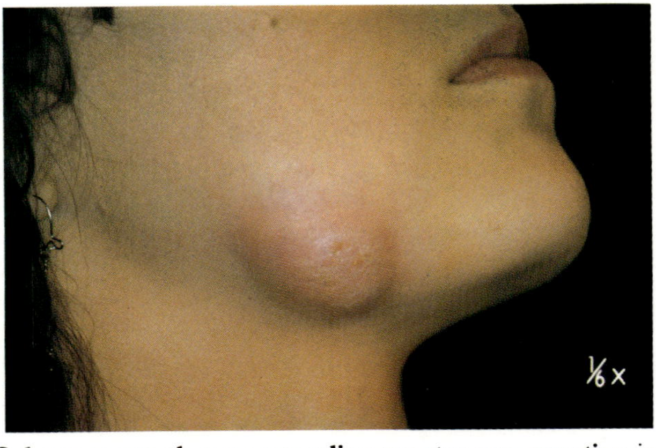

47 Subcutaneous abscess preceding spontaneous eruption in a case of pericoronitis of the lower right wisdom tooth.

treatment for acute inflammatory symptoms. The duration of the pre-operative therapy is usually less than a week. Extraction of the wisdom tooth was preceded in only 2.1% of the cases by the incision of an abscess and in 8.1% by antibiotic treatment. One should keep in mind, however that these figures are based on out-patients only.

3.2.2 Caries and disorders of the pulp

On breaking through the mucous membrane, the wisdom tooth comes under the influence of the oral environment. In principle, therefore, one can observe all the disorders which are found in the other teeth. The incidence of caries is generally high, since the position of the tooth, the formation of a pericoronal pocket and lack of function lead to retention of debris and adherence of plaque (**44**). The high incidence of enamel hypomineralisation and the fact that oral hygiene is made more difficult are both additional caries-disposing factors. Surprisingly, one occasionally finds carious defects in retained teeth when there is no apparent connection with the oral cavity.

Pulp disorders practically always lead to extraction, since amputation or extirpation of the pulp under aseptic conditions is scarcely possible. Equally, root treatment and apicectomy are out of the question on account of the variable conditions of the root canals, the inaccessible location and the fact that the root tips are frequently curved.

3.2.3 Cysts

Both radicular and follicular cysts are observed in wisdom teeth, follicular cysts being more common. If the eruption of the third molar is slow, the dental follicle is continually exposed to infections of many kinds, which may lead to cyst formation. They can develop to considerable size in the ascending ramus and body of the mandible without showing symptoms (**48**) and are often discovered accidentally on a radiograph. They necessitate an operation which includes extraction of the wisdom tooth in addition to cystectomy. The cyst capsule must be examined histopathologically, since other disorders may be connected with cystic changes in this region. In the differential diagnosis, keratocysts and ameloblastomas should be taken into account above everything else.

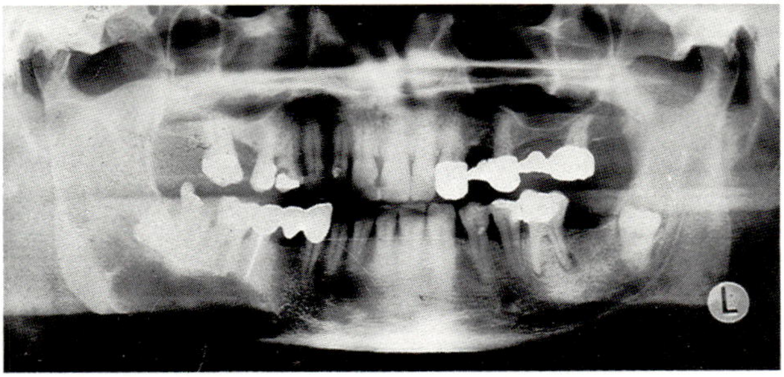

48 Extensive follicular cyst originating in the lower right wisdom tooth.

3.2.4 Suspected tumours

Follicular cysts may give rise to cystic ameloblastomas which clinically and radiographically cannot be differentiated.

Whenever a multilocular lesion is radiologically visible, and is not simulated by the presence of bony ridges, a semi-malignant tumour of this kind is to be suspected (**49**).

A *mucosal ulcer* in the neighbourhood of a completely or partially retained wisdom tooth must be regarded as malignant until this possibility has been excluded (**50, 51**). In rare cases, the epithelium of the dental follicle is the matrix for the formation of carcinomas; their frequency has been estimated by Fröhlich (1952) as 1:100 000. In the case of elongated wisdom teeth which are in contact with the mucous membrane of the opposite jaw, a degeneration is likewise possible as a result of mechanical irritation. If there is the slightest suspicion, the patient should be referred to a specialized clinic which can carry out a biopsy at the

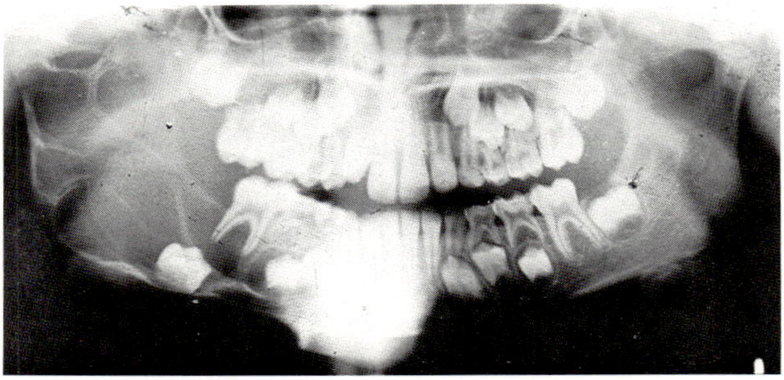

49 Cystic ameloblastoma of the right mandible with displacement of the second molar.

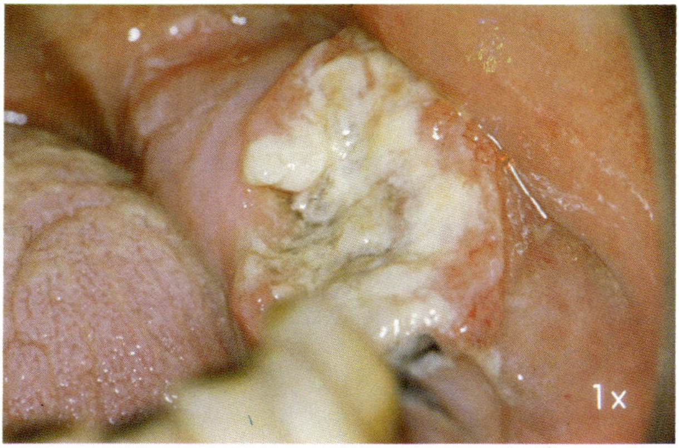

50 Keratinising squamous cell carcinoma in the retromolar triangle.

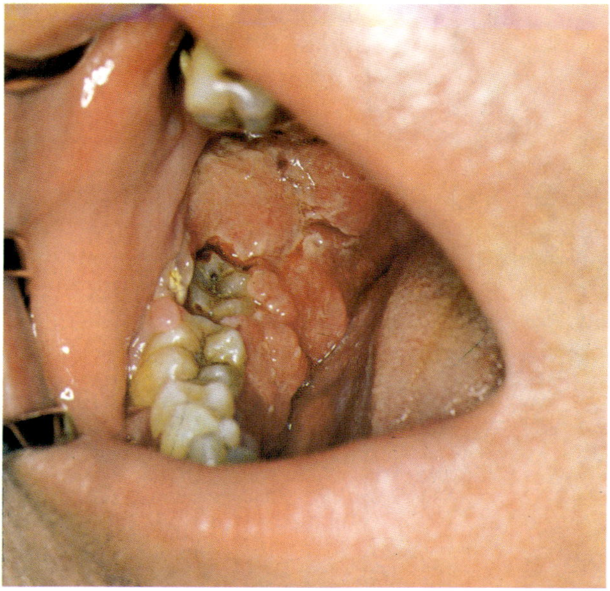

51 Extensive carcinoma in the region of the angle of the right mandible (from the collection of Prof. R. Becker).

same time as the extraction of the wisdom tooth and, if a malignant tumour is found to be present, can undertake further therapy.

3.2.5 Neuralgiform pains

Symptoms of trigeminal neuralgia, otalgia or vague jaw and head pains may all be caused by a retained wisdom tooth. Pains of this sort should be considered grounds for radiological investigation. It sometimes happens that patients are treated in vain for years by different specialists until a wisdom tooth is found to be the cause of the symptoms, and removed. Such phenomena are understandable if the pain is primarily experienced as earache (otalgia) or headache. The extraction of the wisdom teeth should follow even if the connection cannot be established for certain. This also holds for lower wisdom teeth in contact with the inferior alveolar nerve, if inflammation has led to irritation of the nerve.

3.2.6 Focal sepsis

The diagnosis 'focal sepsis' is problematic, since there is no typical picture of a focal disorder. According to Rost (1981), a 'focus' is understood as a chronically diseased region of tissue

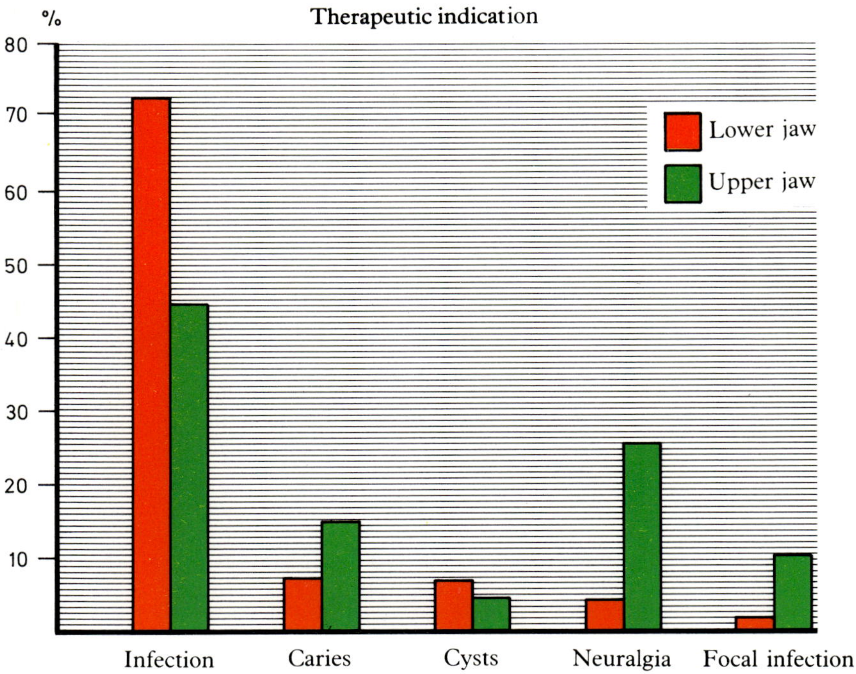

52 Percentage distribution of the therapeutic indications for extraction of the wisdom teeth.

from which general disorders or transferred processes remote from the focus are initiated and maintained in the organism. Thus, teeth are associated with specific organs, the wisdom teeth in particular with the heart or the kidneys.

The significance of a vital retained wisdom tooth as a focus in the presence of a focal disorder or where a focal sepsis is suspected, is controversial. While a connection must be regarded as unlikely in the case of complete retention, it is possible in the case of partly retained teeth with chronically infected pockets. In doubtful cases one must decide on extraction, especially if a regular arrangement in the tooth row is not expected.

The significance of the tooth, mouth and jaw areas in focal disorder has certainly been exaggerated and many teeth removed without good reason; scepticism, therefore, seems to be in order. Above all, the indications for tooth extraction must be reviewed in relation to the fundamental disorder of the patient; e.g. the indications are greater in the case of endocarditis than in a great many skin disorders in which the connection with a dental focus is much less likely.

52 shows the frequency distribution of the above-mentioned disorders as therapeutic indications. Compared with infection, which is the basis for therapeutic tooth extraction in 72.9% of cases in the lower jaw and 44.7% in the upper jaw, all the other indications are of minor significance.

4 SURGICAL PROCEDURE

4.1 Patient preparation

4.1.1 Case history and general examination

The indications and the operation can be influenced in various ways by the general state of health of the patient; a careful case history is therefore essential. We favour a combined written and oral procedure. A relatively simple enquiry form allows the patient to indicate the most important ailments. This form is used as the basis for the oral examination, by means of which the information already given can be brought up to the required level. In the case of insufficient particulars, the doctor in charge should always be contacted. Under the heading of 'general illnesses', after infectious diseases which usually necessitate special safety measures (e.g. tuberculosis, hepatitis), those disorders which influence either the choice of local anaesthetic and its additives, or the surgical procedure, or both, are of special interest. Illnesses which complicate, or even prevent altogether, the inclusion of a vasoconstrictive supplement are especially numerous. The main ones are disorders of cardiac circulation, diabetes mellitus, hyperthyroidism and epilepsy. Since sufficiently deep and long-lasting anaesthesia and a blood-free operating field are desirable during the extraction of a wisdom tooth, one must make a decision on the application of a vasoconstrictive supplement in each individual case. Here again the decision may be facilitated by referring back to the general practitioner or consultant in charge of the case. If the supplement cannot be used, a mepivacaine preparation (Scandicain, Meaverin) should be employed instead, since this local anaesthetic has a certain vasoconstrictive action.

The surgical procedure is affected by haematological disorders, predisposition to haemorrhage, anticoagulant therapy, diabetes mellitus and treatment with corticosteroids, radiotherapy or immunosuppressive drugs. Certain disorders necessitate special preparation or in-patient treatment.

With the medical history there should be a general survey investigation including, after examination and before surgical

Form for taking Case History

Surname____________________First name(s)____________________

Date of birth__________

Address____

____

(1) Are you suffering from any general disorder? yes/no

If yes, give details____________________________________

(2) During the last 2 years, have you been a hospital in-patient or been under medical treatment? yes/no

If yes, give details____________________________________

(3) Are you taking any form of regular medication? yes/no

If yes, give details____________________________________

(4) Are you pregnant? yes/no

(5) Do you suffer from any of the following disorders? yes/no

If yes, state which____________________________________

Cardiac disease	Circulatory disorders
Blood disorders	Liver disease
Allergies	Kidney disease
Thyroid disorders	Epilepsy
Lung disease	Intestinal disorders
Nervous disorders	

(6) Are you prone to haemorrhages or bruising? yes/no

Date Signature

intervention, measurement of heart rate and blood pressure (Tetsch and Wagner, 1979). In many cases, a previously unsuspected hypertension is discovered, which should be clarified and treated by a specialist. Similarly, close observation of the patient while the case history is being taken often gives useful information about the general condition.

4.1.2 Patient information and declaration of consent

Following diagnosis, the situation must be explained to the patient. The necessity for the operation, the procedure and the most serious complications should be pointed out. A comprehensive explanation of *all possible complications* is increasingly encouraged. This is an inappropriate requirement and leads to a considerable feeling of insecurity in the patient. Before a routine operation, where there is a high probability that there will be no complications, the information should cover the post-operative swelling, inability to work, restricted ability to drive and problems related to nutrition (Table 7). Further explanations are necessary after the operation; these are given in Section 4.7.

Table 7 Content of the explanatory discussion

Explanation of the diagnostic findings
Necessity for the operation
Alternative types of therapy
Surgical procedure
Possible complications
Restricted ability to drive

In special situations, a detailed pre-operative explanation is necessary. These are: danger of damage to nerves because of possible contact of the root with the inferior dental canal; expected sinus complications and all pathological processes which are associated with retained wisdom teeth and are treated by extraction.

Aderhold and Frenkel (1981) discuss a comprehensive written pre-operative explanation which, together with the discussion with the dentist, serves as the basis for obtaining written consent and in the case of minors must be undersigned by the parent or guardian.

Patient Information Form
(Modified after Aderhold and Frenkel, 1981)

For any treatment, the consent of the patient and, in the case of minors, of the legally responsible adult, must be obtained. This leaflet contains important information which, if you wish, will be further explained by the surgeon in charge.

Illness

If the correct arrangement of the dentition is not achieved by the normal eruption of the teeth, or if parts of teeth remain in the jaw, serious and constantly recurring inflammation can occur, which may possibly have a considerable effect on the general state of health. There is the additional possibility of damage to other teeth and the surrounding tissue. The teeth or parts of teeth should therefore be extracted.

Surgical procedure

Surgical extraction of teeth or parts of tooth embedded in the jaw proceeds through their exposure by folding back the mucous membrane and partially removing the portion of jaw bone which surrounds the tooth. This operation is carried out while you are under local anaesthesia. To avoid general complications, you are asked about previous ailments. Tell the surgeon all the illnesses that you have had, or which you are suffering from at present and state what medications you take regularly. There are seldom any complications with local anaesthetic. Please ask if you would like more information.

On the day of the operation you will not be able to drive. Therefore you should be accompanied to the appointment and not drive a vehicle yourself.

On the first day after surgery, there will be swelling in the region of the operation, which responds well to tepid poultices. You will receive advice concerning the operation as well as special information about conditions following surgery and eventual medication.

No surgeon can give an absolute guarantee about the course of the treatment, since every operation has risks. Wound infection and bleeding are possible complications. After the operation you will be informed about the necessary precautionary measures.

In the lower jaw the teeth lie very close to the nerves of the tongue, lower jaw and lower lip. In rare cases, these nerves may be damaged, even with the most careful surgery. According to the extent of the damage, there are differing degrees of loss of sensation in the area supplied by the nerve, which in rare cases may persist for months or be permanent.

In the upper jaw the teeth are partly adjacent to the sinus cavity. If, during the operation, this cavity is penetrated, the wound will be tightly closed. You are informed about this because in these cases special procedures must be observed.

Only the most important complications can be mentioned here. There is in addition a series of rare risks, which your surgeon will be pleased to explain if you so wish.

Special circumstances which occur during an operation may necessitate an alteration of the operation or further surgery. Give your consent to this also, or you will have the additional inconvenience, if the operation is discontinued, of having to have it completed later.

The explanatory discussion
In this leaflet we have given you the information which, in medical experience, is essential. The surgeon who examines you will inform you about the results of the investigation in the discussion which will follow and will ask for your signature on the consent form. If there is something which you have not understood, or if you wish to have more details, please ask about anything you consider important.

Declaration of consent

Mr/Ms_____________ has held an explanatory discussion with me today. Following an explanation of my illness and the possible consequences, the scope and planned course of the treatment and its aim were described to me in a form which I could understand. The typical risks were explained to me. I realise that the surgeon and his team can give no guarantee for the success of the operation.

Following a discussion of alternative methods of treatment, I have decided in favour of the planned operation:_____________________

____

____

____

I hereby declare that I agree to this and to any extension or alteration which may become necessary during the course of the operation. Follow-up investigations which may possibly be necessary, and the medically recommended procedure for the period after the operation have been made known to me.

I confirm that I have had sufficient time to ask any questions of interest to me and to reach my decision concerning the consent to the operation.

Supplements:_________________________________

____

Place:_______________________________________

Date:____

Surgeon:_____________________________________

Patient:_____________________________________

Witness:_____________________________________

4.1.3 Local preparation

Widely differing opinions exist concerning the effectiveness of pre-surgical oral disinfection. Flushing with anti-bacterial solutions before a wisdom tooth operation is not necessary, since only a minimal bacterial reduction is achieved (Sonntag and Werner, 1981). *Disinfection* of the oral mucosa is impossible and should not therefore be attempted; in addition to damaging the mucosa, it can lead to bacterial selection. Neither does disinfection of the skin around the mouth produce a noticeable effect. Of course, it is essential in extra-oral operations.

On the other hand, removal of calculus and plaque before the operation is recommended, since infection may set in on account of the close proximity of the wound to the second molar, or through calculus being dislodged into the extraction wound. It is advisable to carry out a thorough cleaning of the teeth at least 24 hours before the operation.

4.1.4 Premedication

The aims of premedication may be divided into central sedation, control of the sympathetic tone, central control of pain and reduction of the risk of infection.

For *over-anxious patients,* central sedation is advisable, as it is for children who resist treatment and arteriosclerotic patients, and in cases of anxiety-induced pain or tendency to hyperventilation.

Among psycho-sedative medications, hypnotics and tranquillisers are suitable for dental practice (e.g. Luminaletten, Valium, 5-10 mg). It is advisable to treat pale, hypotensive adolescents and hypotensive patients with a tendency to collapse with a sympathomimetic (Effortil, Norvadral). As a precautionary measure, the operation should be carried out with the patient lying down. After the operation he should be returned to a standing position very slowly to reduce the risk of an orthostatic collapse.

Antibiotic coverage is only necessary as a prophylactic measure in cases where the resistance is lowered (i.e. corticosteroid treatment, chemotherapy, radiotherapy, leukaemic diseases, heart valve replacements, endocarditis, rheumatic fever, drastically compromised general state of health) and if the results of infection are expected to be dangerous or if there is a high risk of local infection. It is hardly ever necessary in dental practice and even in the hospital it is the exception rather than the rule.

4.1.5 Anaesthesia

As a rule, the wisdom tooth operation can be carried out under *local* anaesthesia. If all four teeth are to be extracted, it is advisable to take out the teeth in two separate sittings, extracting only the antagonists unilaterally. In this way the masticatory function of one side is ensured and the problem of bilateral anaesthesia is avoided. Simultaneous bilateral anaesthesia of the lingual nerve can lead to disturbance of the swallowing process due to lack of co-ordination and even to aspiration. Blocking of the inferior alveolar nerve and the buccal nerve in the lower jaw (**53**) and the posterior superior alveolar nerve and the greater palatine nerve in the upper jaw (**54, 55**) is undertaken. The addition of a vasoconstrictor is recommended in order to obtain sufficiently deep and long-lasting anaesthesia and to provide a relatively blood-free operating field, so that the view is not obscured.

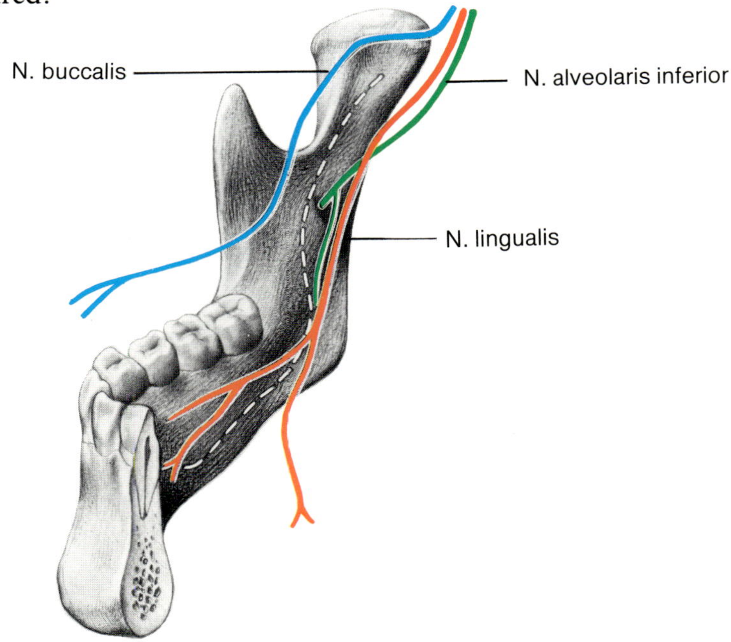

53 Nerve supply to the mandible.

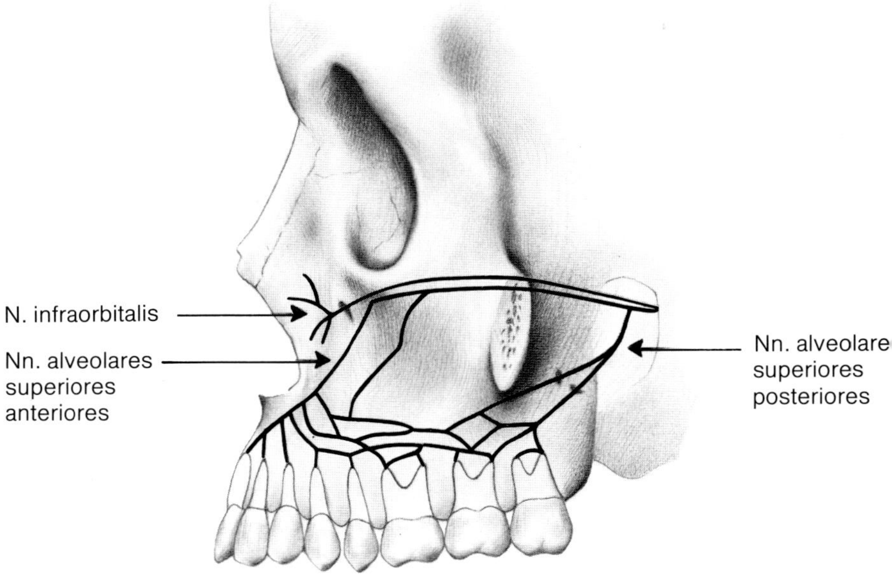

54 Nerve supply to the upper jaw (vestibular view).

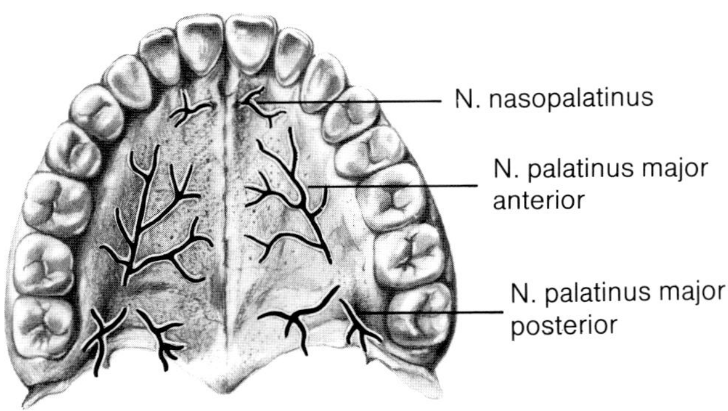

55 Nerve supply to the upper jaw (palatal aspect).

Local anaesthetics can be divided into p-amino benzoic acid esters and anilides (amide aliphatic carbonic acids) (Table 8). The *ester-type* anaesthetics (e.g. Tetracain, Pantocain, Gingicain) are used as topical anaesthetics and these days are only applied as infiltration anaesthetics in dental practice in cases of chronic liver disease, since they are broken down in the blood and tissues by

Anaesthetic	Concentration (%)	Vasoconstrictive supplement	Concentration of vasoconstrictor	Limiting dose local anaesthetic (mg/kg)	Maximum permissible dose (ml) 20 kg	70 kg
Benzoic acid esters						
Procaine (novocain)	2	—	—	7	7.0	24.0
	2	adrenalin	1:20 000	14	1.4	5.0
	2	adrenalin	1:200 000	14	14.0	49.0
Anilide						
Lidocaine	2	—	—	3	2.8	10.0
(Xylocain, Xylestesin)	2	adrenalin	1:50 000	7	3.5	12.5
	2	noradrenalin	1:25 000	3	1.7	6.2
	2	adrenalin + noradrenalin	1:25 000 1:25 000		1.7	6.2
Mepivacaine	2	—	—	3	2.8	10.0
(Scandicain, Meaverin)	3	—	—	1.5	1.0	3.5
	2	adrenalin	1:66 000	7	4.7	16.5
	2	noradrenalin	1:25 000	7	1.7	6.2
	2	noradrenalin	1:40 000	3	2.0	7.0
Butanilicaine	2	—	—	1.5	1.0	3.5
(Hostacain)	2	noradrenalin	1:25 000	7	1.7	6.2
	3	noradrenalin	1:25 000	3	1.7	6.2
Carticain	4	adrenalin	1:200 000	7	3.5	12.0
(Ultracain DS, DS forte)	4	adrenalin	1:100 000	7	3.5	12.0
Bupivacain	0.5	—	—	1	4.0	14.0
(Carbostesin)	0.25	—	—	1		
	0.5	adrenalin	1:200 000	2	8.0	28.0
	0.25	adrenalin	1:200 000	2	16.0	56.0

The maximum permissible doses given in ml are calculated on the basis of the limiting doses of both the local anaesthetic and of the vasoconstrictive supplement.

esterases and do not cause a strain on the liver. As a breakdown product, in addition to diethyl amino ethanol, a benzene ring with a p-amino group is formed. These 'para substances' frequently give rise to allergies, with which 1–2% of the patients treated with procaine are afflicted. 5% of allergics and 9% of people with a contact dermatitis show an allergic reaction to procaine (Weber, 1981). Skin manifestations predominate in cases of procaine allergy. The quicker the appearance of the first symptom, the earlier will be the onset of the possibly fatal anaphylactic shock.

p-Hydroxybenzoic acid methyl esters are also added to other anaesthetic solutions (anilides) as a preservative against bacterial contamination. Only in the early days were anaesthetics produced without additives of this sort. They can be ordered from the manufacturers if they are not on the market. Their use is absolutely recommended if the patient is known to suffer from 'para-group allergy'. If there is any suspicion of an allergy against a local anaesthetic a skin specialist who is familiar with problems of this type should be consulted.

The most widely used local anaesthetics are the *anilides* (amide type). They possess a certain vasodilatory action in addition to the anaesthetic effect. The sole exception is mepivacaine (Scandicain, Meaverin), which has vasoconstrictive properties and so can be used if, on the grounds of the general state of health, a vasoconstrictive additive must be avoided.

The tolerance dose is reduced by the use of high concentration solutions (3%, 4%). It is recommended that in these cases, and also with extremes of weight, the individually permissible limiting dose should be determined.

In Table 8 the maximum values for 20 kg and 70 kg patients are given. When treating children, the maximum dose of many preparations is insufficient to achieve sufficiently deep anaesthesia; the simultaneous application of a topical anaesthetic reduces the limiting dosage of the infiltration anaesthetic.

Adrenalin and *noradrenalin* are the most important vasoconstrictors. In addition to providing a relatively blood-free operating field, they increase the depth and duration of anaesthesia and reduce the toxicity of the anaesthetic by delaying its removal. A subordinate role is played by octapressin, which has a smaller vasoconstrictive effect and which is contra-indicated during pregnancy on account of its labour-inducing properties.

The *catecholamines* are pharmacologically extremely active substances, which exhibit a high toxicity if they are rapidly absorbed in unphysiological doses. This can lead, with inadvertent intravenous injections, to complications *even at lower doses*. In the case of anaesthesia by injection in the lower jaw, puncture of a blood vessel is to be expected in 10% of cases. The risk of an intravenous injection can only be reduced to a minimum by consistent aspiration at each injection.

It is not widely known that the vasoconstrictive supplement can also be a limiting factor for the amount of anaesthetic solution which can be injected. In the case of adrenalin, the maximum dose is 0.25 mg for adults and 0.15 mg for children. The problem of local anaesthesia for high-risk patients is considered in Chapter 7. General anaesthesia is only necessary in rare and exceptional circumstances, such as:

- blood clotting disorders,
- local infections,
- allergy to all local anaesthetics,
- uncooperative patients.

Severe *clotting disorders* are responsible for extensive haematomas if a blood vessel is damaged during anaesthesia, which can lead to mechanical hindrance of breathing and a life-endangering situation, especially following anaesthesia of the lower jaw.

Local infections may likewise forbid local anaesthesia if the injection must be carried out near the infected area. An extensive anaesthesia is not achieved because of the change in pH of the tissue. There is also the danger of transfer of infection and the possible occurrence of sepsis as a serious complication.

A local infection is therefore treated in the first instance and the surgical extraction of the tooth follows as the acute symptoms subside. If the formation of focal abscesses necessitates an incision under general anaesthesia, this operation may be combined with the extraction of the wisdom teeth.

Rarely, there is an *allergy* to all the available local anaesthetics. In these cases the operation must be carried out under general anaesthesia.

There is a further indication in the case of *uncooperative patients*, including the mentally retarded, who cannot be treated under local anaesthesia (Kleemann *et al.*, 1981).

The following conditions must be fulfilled in carrying out dental treatment under *general anaesthesia*:

- adequate equipment,
- adequate training,

- surgeon not doubling as anaesthetist,
- control over complications,
- adequate post-anaesthesia supervision,
- adequate balance between anaesthetic risk and indications for surgical operation.

As a rule, the delivery of general anaesthesia is under the control of an anaesthetist. Of the various procedures of general anaesthesia, intubation anaesthesia is advised for intra-oral surgery. In addition to the ease of management breathing is not obstructed, and aspiration is prevented by the endotracheal tube and by a throat pack.

4.2 Instrumentation

Special handpieces which exhibit numerous advantages have been developed for surgical use: they ensure adequate sterility by

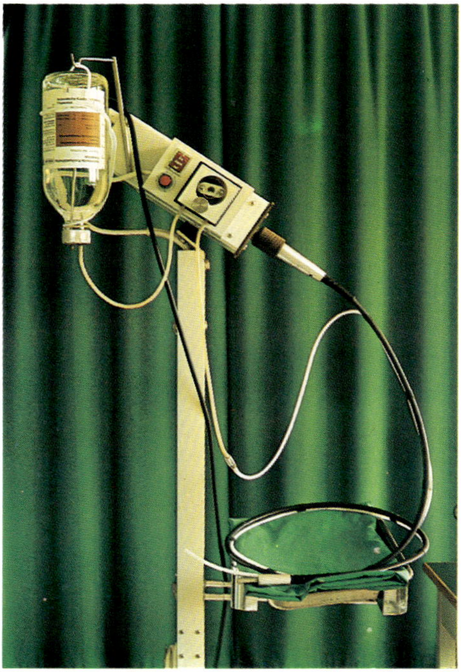

56 Surgical unit (made by Aesculap) with automatic supply of sterile physiological saline by means of a pump.

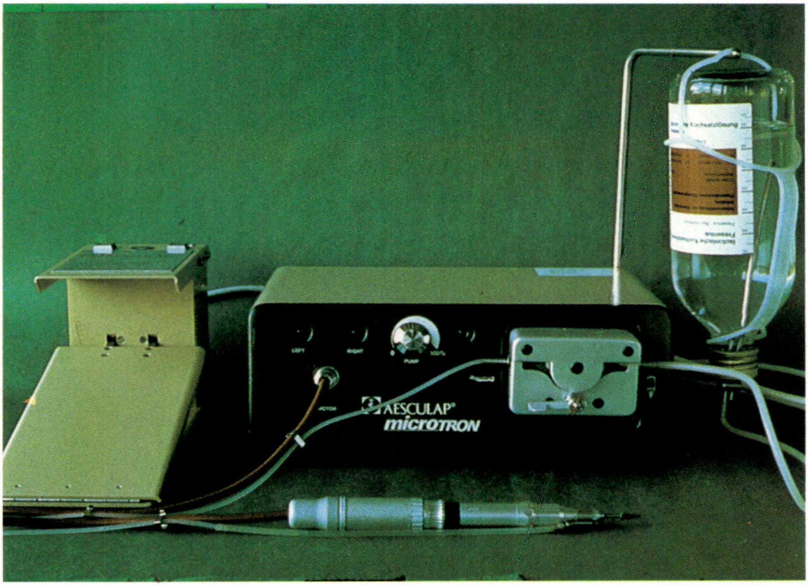

57 Surgical unit (made by Aesculap) with automatic supply of sterile physiological saline by means of a pump.

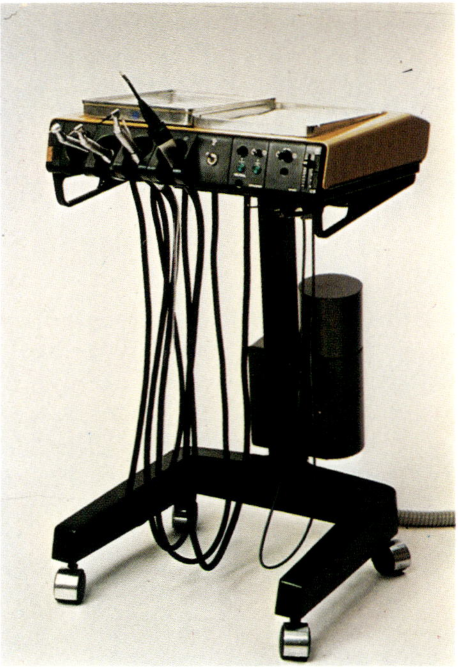

58 Dental treatment unit (Sirodont, made by Siemens) with option for physiological saline.

employing removable and sterilisable drive shafts and, through special attachments, offer the advantage of automatic supply of physiological saline. In addition, they possess high torque at low speeds and therefore facilitate osteotomy (**56**). Indeed the purchase of a machine of this sort for dental practices in which operations are regularly carried out makes sense (**57, 58**).

A high efficiency vacuum suction circuit and an electrotome are essential requirements for trouble-free operations.

Disposable instruments should be used as far as possible. Syringes, injection needles, scalpels, suction tubes, drapes and atraumatic sutures are obtainable in this form (**59**).

The standard instrument set for the extraction of wisdom teeth consists of:

- Drapes
- Drape fasteners
- Suction tube
- Artery clamps
- Dental mirror
- Dental probe
- Forceps (dental, surgical, anatomical)
- Langenbeck wound retractor
- Scalpel
- Periosteal elevator
- Handpiece
- Round burs
- Lindemann burs
- Straight elevators
- Claw elevators
- Wisdom tooth forceps
- Bayonet forceps
- Sharp curette
- Rongeurs
- Needle holder
- Atraumatic sutures
- Scissors (dissection, thread)
- Luniatschek pack applicators
- Bite swabs

For special situations additional instruments may be necessary (e.g. calculus-removing instruments for the extraction of small root fragments, forceps for the removal of tooth fragments from the sinus). Absolute sterility of the whole instrument set is an obvious requirement. It is recommended that the tray system, which has proved useful in the whole field of surgery, be used.

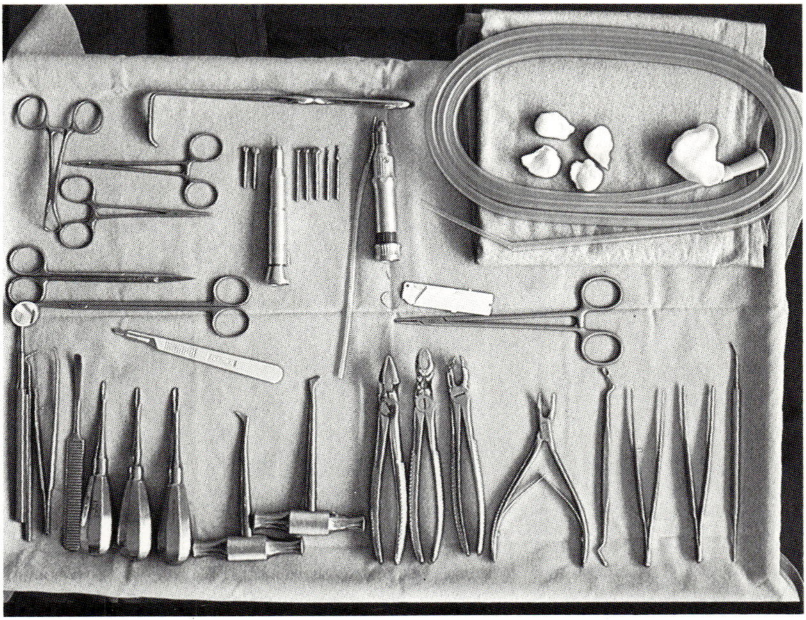

59 Standard instrument set for operative extraction of wisdom teeth.

4.3 Preparation of the surgical team

Surgical disinfection of the hands

The surgical disinfection of the hands should kill off foreign and adherent bacteria. Persistent absence of bacteria is not achieved, however, since the micro-organisms of the deep layers of the skin pass to the surface with the sweat. Surgical hand disinfection is essential for all operations with the exception of a straightforward tooth extraction.

Many quick-acting disinfectants which produce sufficient disinfection with a washing time of 5 minutes are available. Since hands and forearms must be disinfected up to the elbows, short-sleeved shirts should be worn. The first step is the preliminary wash with water and liquid soap and cleaning of the fingernails with sterile brushes. Hands and forearms are dried with a disposable towel and finally rubbed together for 5 minutes with 2 × 5 ml of the disinfectant solution (e.g. Primasept-M, Braunol, Braunisan, Desderman, Frekasept 80, Sterillium).

Soap and disinfectant should be obtained from a wall dispenser which can be operated with the foot or elbow. Finally, the hands are again dried with a sterile disposable towel.

Protective clothing

Surgical cap and mask are put on before the surgical scrub. Afterwards the protective clothing is completed with a sterile gown and rubber gloves. This is especially important in practices where several operations are carried out one after the other, because then the surgical scrub has only to be undergone once.

4.4 Incision

4.4.1 General aspects

Disposable scalpels should be used for the incision (e.g. Feather disposable scalpels No. 15). The incision must be appropriate for the particular situation and results from the pre-operative planning. Basically, the following general conditions need to be fulfilled when raising a mucoperiosteal flap:

- no damage to important anatomical structures,
- a good view of the operating field,
- sufficient blood supply to the mucoperiosteal flap (a wide base to the flap),
- possibility of enlarging the incision,
- wound suture on intact bony support,
- favourable scar formation.

Of all the possible types of incision, the angled incision has proved the most suitable for the extraction of wisdom teeth in both upper and lower jaws.

4.4.2 Incision in the lower jaw

The anatomical situation in the region of the angle of the jaw, with the close proximity of the course of the lingual nerve, must be considered when making the incision. In general, *angled incisions* with a distal leg on the ascending mandibular ramus and vestibular extension to the level of the second molar have proved successful.

The profession shows an increasing number of cases of *damage to the lingual nerve* following surgical wisdom tooth extraction (Scheunemann and Hausamen, 1980). This is a very unpleasant complication, since disturbances of sensation and unilateral disturbance of taste may lead to a considerable subjective handicap for the patient. Damage is possible through anaesthesia as well as through incision. In individual cases the cause is difficult to establish retrospectively. Since direct injury to the nerve during anaesthesia must be considered a very rare occurrence, according to the studies of Schulz (1981), injury due to a haematoma or to iatrogenic operative damage are probably the most frequent causes. Not uncommonly, the course of the scar shows that an incorrect or hazardous incision line was chosen. The ascending ramus diverges laterally to a widely differing extent in different individuals (**60**). All incisions which

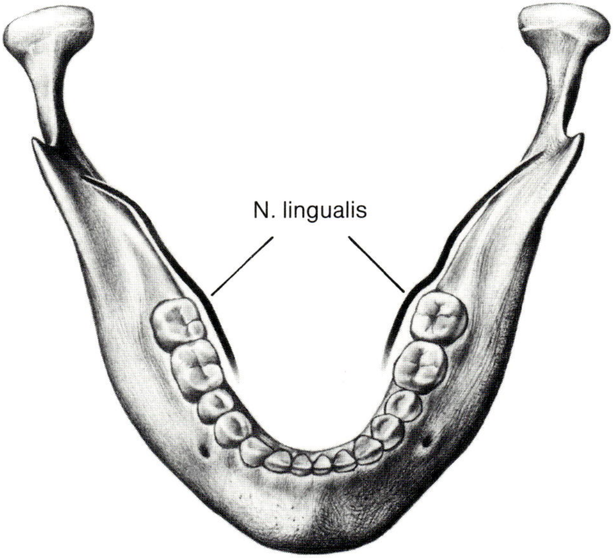

60 Divergence of the ascending mandibular ramus and relationship to the lingual nerve.

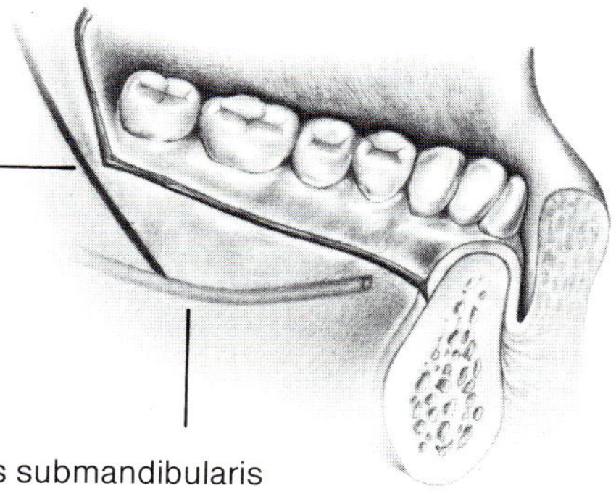

61 Lingual view of the lower jaw, showing the lingual nerve and the submandibular duct.

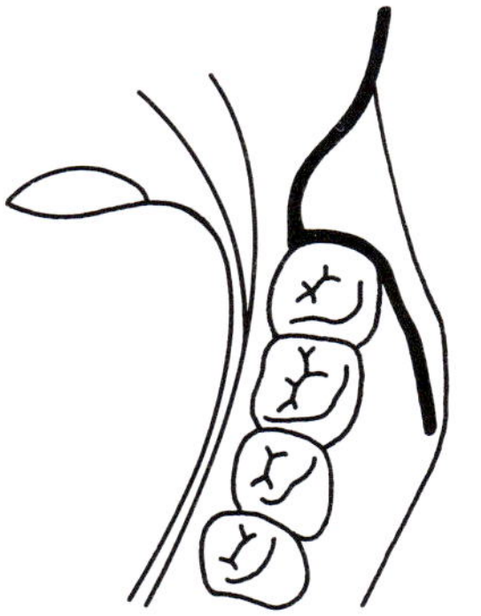

62 Incision for surgical extraction of a lower wisdom tooth.

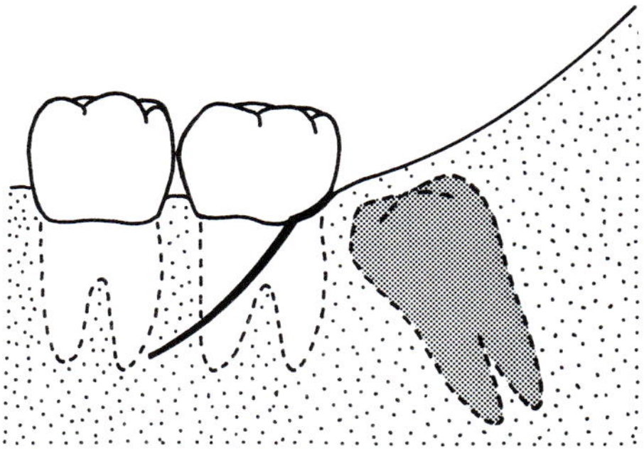

63 Vestibular incision for surgical extraction of a lower wisdom tooth.

are made along the occlusal plane distal to the second molars carry the risk of damage to the lingual nerve, which in this region lies on the surface below the mucous membrane. It passes, as does the inferior alveolar nerve, between the two pterygoid muscles, down the medial side of the internal maxillary artery and hence can lie anterior and medial to the inferior alveolar nerve. It runs beside the medial pterygoid muscle and the ascending ramus, posterior to the retromolar triangle, for a short distance, close above the periosteum, under the mucosa beside the lower wisdom tooth, first over the submandibular gland (**61**) then over the mylohyoid muscle to the lateral border of the tongue and finally to the outer surface of the hyoglossal muscle.

The incision for extraction of lower wisdom teeth can *safely* be made on the lateral anterior edge of the ascending ramus, i.e. on a bony support. It is assumed that the surgeon will previously have established the anatomical situation by palpation. The incision is carried from the lateral margin to the distolingual cusp of the last molar. This distal arm should be about 2 cm long; if necessary it can be extended on to the ascending ramus. Bleeding from the buccal artery, which occasionally occurs, can be stopped with clamps and coagulation of the vessel. By making a bow-shaped incision, one can ensure that the final closure will lie at least partially on a bony support (**62**).

With all types of retention which have resulted in contact of the last two molars, this incision will be made through the marginal periodontium of the second molar. It must always be extended in a vestibular direction. It starts there in the distal third of the marginal periodontium of the lower second molar and is continued in a diagonal arc mesially and caudally for a distance of 1–2 cm (**63**). This incision results in a triangular flap with a broad base on the vestibular side and ensures an adequate blood supply and a good view of the operation field.

The marginal periodontium can be preserved if a distoangular retention is present or if, in other forms of retention, there is no contact with the last molars (**64**).

Following the incision, which should in the first instance be taken as far as the bony substratum, the mucoperiosteal flap is raised by inserting a periosteal elevator into the medial arm of the cut. Any overgrowth by the dental follicle or by formation of granular tissue as a result of previous inflammation is sectioned

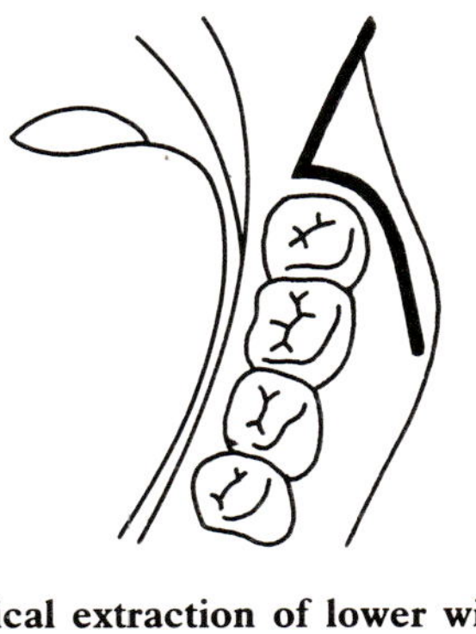

64 Incision for surgical extraction of lower wisdom teeth, showing preservation of the marginal periodontium of the second molar.

with a scalpel or dissecting scissors. The periosteum is not damaged by this procedure. The flap is pushed back sufficiently far to allow a Langenbeck retractor to be inserted between the flap and the lateral surface of the lower jaw and held there without using force.

4.4.3 Incision in the upper jaw

The *angled incision* is also utilised in the upper jaw. There is less danger of causing damage here, since no large blood vessels or nerves pass through the immediate neighbourhood of the wisdom teeth. The distal incision can be made as an extension of the line of the tooth row on to the tuberosity and, as in the lower jaw, can be extended in a vestibular direction with either preservation or inclusion of the marginal periodontium (**65, 66**). Since this is a very inaccessible area the operation field should be prepared on a large scale. In every wisdom tooth extraction in the upper jaw a possible perforation of the antrum must be reckoned with. Should a tooth or a root be displaced into the antrum, access can be enlarged by extension of the vestibular incision, so that the removal of the tooth or tooth fragment as well as the closure of the defect can be carried out with relative ease.

Often, primary incision as far as the bony substratum is problematical in the region of the tuberosity, since an extremely thick – even fibroma-like – layer of soft tissue is not infrequently

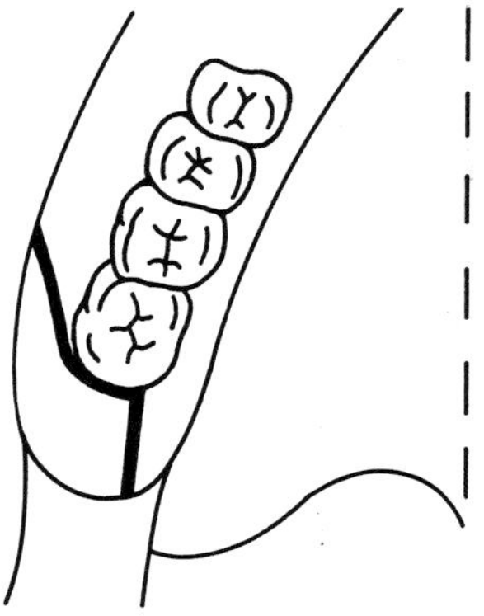

65 Incision for surgical extraction of upper wisdom teeth.

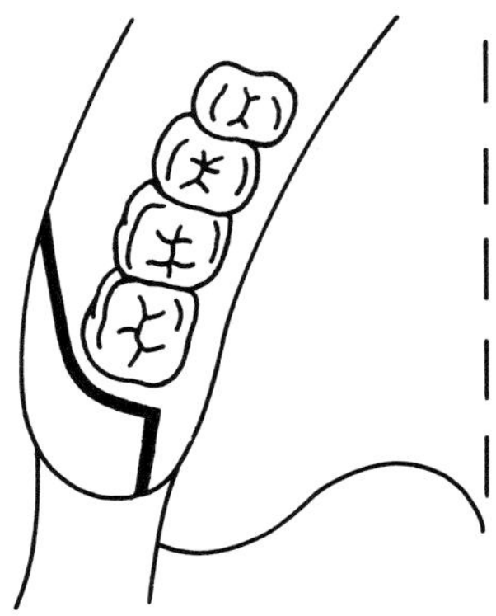

66 Incision in the upper jaw with preservation of the marginal periodontium of the second molar.

found here. A wedge-shaped excision in these cases makes later prosthetic treatment easier.

The standard incision procedure described is modified in individual cases where fistulas, incision wounds, damaged mucous membrane, scars and incisions for teeth not being operated on have to be taken into consideration. If another molar is to be extracted at the same time, the incision should be made so as to include that region of the alveolus as well. If the wisdom tooth and the first molar on one side have to be extracted, marginal incision is recommended.

4.5 Osteotomy

Generally two procedures for tooth extraction are possible: *bone reduction* and the *additional sectioning of the tooth.*

For *bone reduction* the following conditions should be observed:

- the crown of the tooth must be freed at its greatest circumference,
- bone obstructing the path of elevation must be removed,
- a fulcrum must be prepared for support of an elevator.

In each individual case it must be decided whether by division of the tooth the operation can be carried out conservatively and with less damage to the bone.

After exposure of the bone, the bone over the occlusal surface of the tooth crown is removed; the exposure of the vestibular coronal surface follows. Round burs of various sizes or bone chisels are suitable for this procedure.

4.5.1 Instrumentation

We favour *mechanical reduction,* in which the bone is cut out at low speed and must be constantly flushed and cooled with sterile physiological saline. 'Dry cutting' leads to a considerable rise in temperature which lies above that at which albumin coagulates and results in thermal damage to the bone with corresponding disturbance of wound healing (Lentrodt and Bull, 1974, 1976; Tetsch, 1974; Tetsch and Schneider, 1977).

The extent of damage depends upon the rate of revolution, the pressure applied, the size and sharpness of the bur and the structure of the bony tissue. Physiological saline can be supplied via a disposable syringe of suitable size and a blunt cannula. Automatic irrigation, supplied by a pump in a machine which has been specially developed for surgery is better adapted to the purpose. Nowadays, systems are also available for regular dental units which enable the automatic introduction of physiological saline. A pre-selector switch on the unit enables one to choose between a water wash for tooth preparation and saline solution (see **58**). Tapwater – even if made bacteria-free by the use of sterile filters – is not suitable for surgical operations, since as a result of the concentration gradient and corresponding osmotic processes electrolyte depletion can arise in the bone and may possibly cause damage.

Low speed sterilisable *hand-pieces* should be employed. They should be capable of being dismantled easily in order to facilitate cleaning after use. Cleaning with special sprays, as frequently recommended, is inadequate for surgery. Ideally, the arbour or system of tubing leading to the hand-piece should be changed and sterilised after every operation. If this is not possible, as a

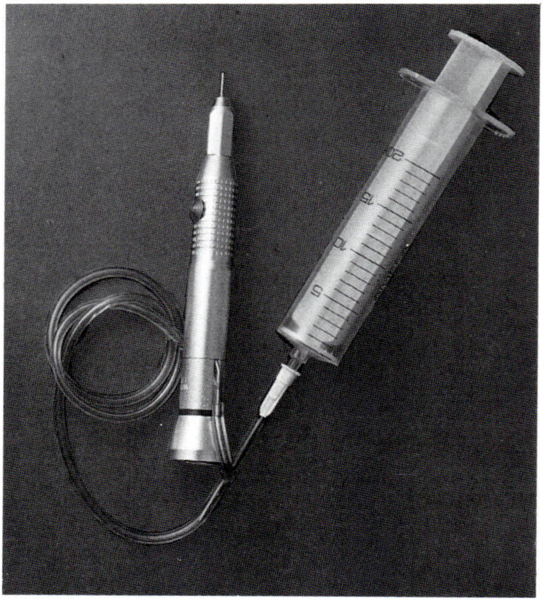

67 Internally cooled hand-piece with system of tubing and disposable syringe (after Kirschner *et al.*).

compromise solution the supply tube should be equipped with a sterile cover and renewed before each operation.

A further development is the *internal cooling system* devised by Kirschner *et al.* (1975, 1976). Sterile physiological saline is led by means of a cannula through the straight or contra-angle handpiece into the bur (**67, 68**). The rinsing solution then runs out of the tip of the instrument and produces superb cooling and at the same time a convenient flushing effect. The use of an internally cooled machine of this type is above all essential if the bur or drill has to be sunk below the surface of the bone (e.g. in forming a furrow in the bone, preparation of a cavity for an endosteal implant or a transplantation). In these procedures, cooling of the surface of the bone is not usually sufficient to prevent a critical rise in temperature in the depths of the bony tissue. In addition, satisfactory results with regard to post-operative complications following wisdom tooth extraction have been reported (Tetsch and Schneider, 1977).

4.5.2 Osteotomy in the lower jaw

The surgical extraction of impacted wisdom teeth can be achieved by *vestibular* or *lingual osteotomy*. While the vestibular route is followed in German clinics, in England the principle of

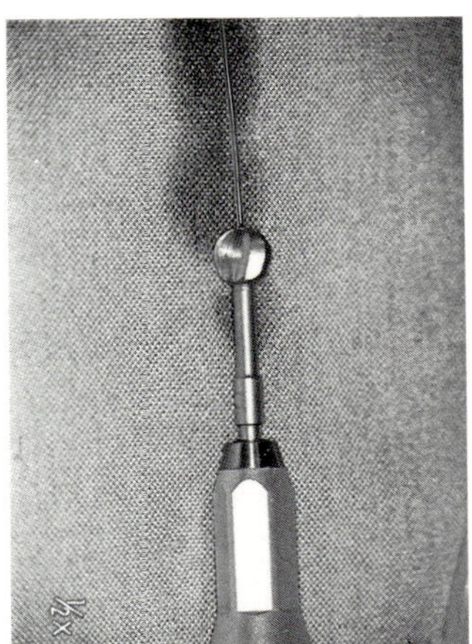

68 Internally cooled bur (made by Aesculap). Physiological saline flows from the working end of the instrument.

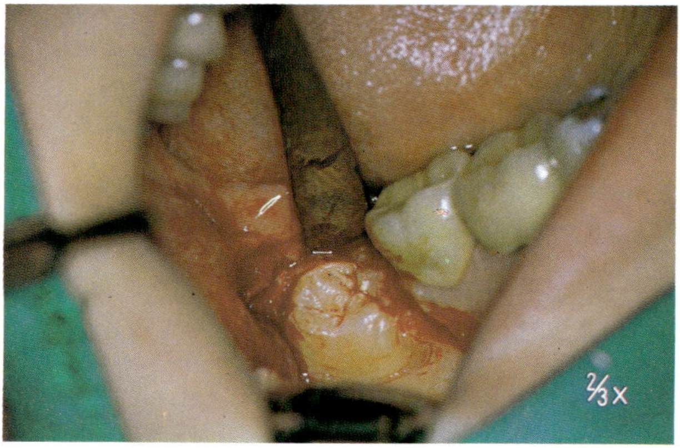

69 Situation after exposure of a vertically retained lower right wisdom tooth. Protection of the lingual soft tissues with a raspatory.

'lingual bone splitting' was introduced by Fry (1933) and James (1933) and in the last few decades developed further by Ward (1956), Killey and Kay (1965) and Rud (1970). The advantages are seen above all in sparing and easy work with only limited bone damage, as the lingual cortical plate is only half as thick as the buccal.

Comparative studies on surgical techniques by Strukmeier and Pape (1950) have shown that in the first two post-operative days following lingual osteotomy serious disturbances occur. They are heralded by swelling in the region of the floor of the mouth. On

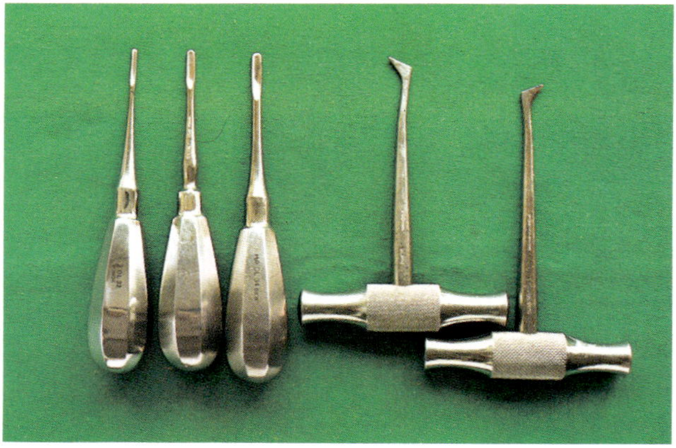

70 Various straight elevators (after Bein) and **claw elevators** (after Winter).

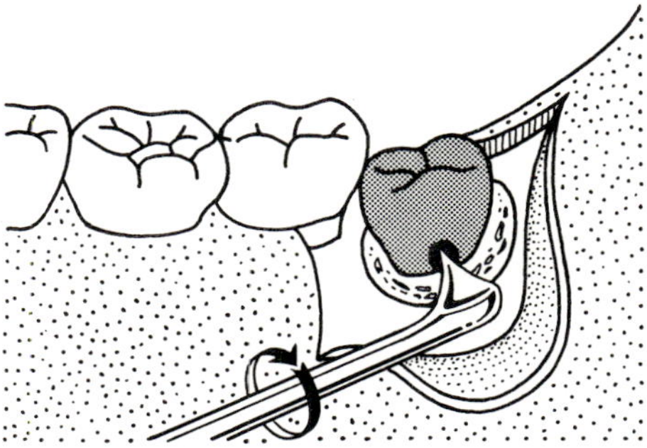

71 Surgical procedure for extraction of a lower vertically impacted wisdom tooth. After exposure of the crown, preparation of an interradicular hole with a bur and luxation of the tooth in a cranial direction using a claw elevator.

the other hand, the vestibular route leads to marked swelling of the cheek and increased problems of wound healing; a careful selection of technique according to the particular situation is recommended. Mesiobuccally impacted wisdom teeth can more easily be extracted from the buccal side; distoangularly, horizontally and deep vertically impacted teeth from the lingual side. Nevertheless, this assumes that the operation is being carried out by a skilled surgeon.

The *hazard* of the lingual procedure lies in the possibility of damage to the lingual nerve. This can be reduced by careful subperiosteal preparation and with sufficient shielding of the soft tissue of the floor of the mouth by means of suitable wound retractors (**69**). Even so, the risk is certainly greater than with

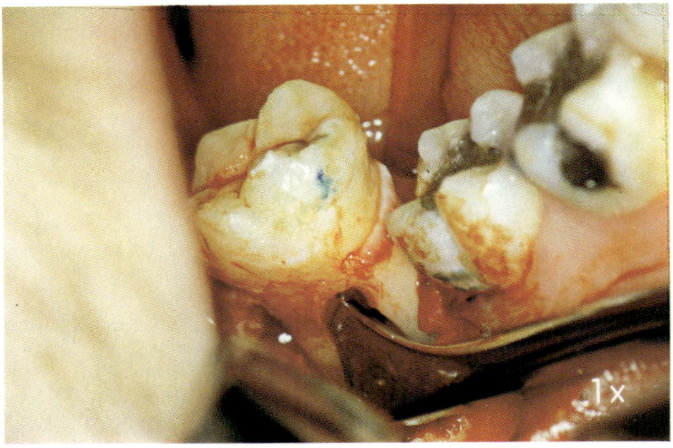

72 Vertical elevation of lower right wisdom tooth with a claw elevator.

vestibular osteotomy and the vestibular access route therefore seems more suitable to us. This is especially true for clinics in which the extraction of wisdom teeth is carried out by junior colleagues and by students as part of a surgical course. This does not exclude the possibility that, in certain particular cases – especially with linguo-angular transverse or inclined retention – the lingual access route may be suitable for an experienced operator.

Vertical retention

As a rule, extraction of vertically retained wisdom teeth presents no problems if there are no root abnormalities. Following vestibular exposure of the crown, an interradicular insertion point is made with a small round Lindemann bur and the tooth luxated cranially using a claw elevator (**70**), which is supported using the relatively stable vestibular cortical plate as a fulcrum (**71, 72**). This procedure is without doubt the least hazardous, since no damage to the neighbouring teeth and no fracture of the mandible can occur.

The insertion of *elevators* is essential for the extraction of impacted teeth, as they cannot be grasped with forceps. However, elevators should be used with the greatest care because there is the possible danger of damaging or luxating adjacent teeth, fracturing the jaw or the alveolar process, damaging soft tissues, puncturing the sinus or displacing roots into the inferior dental canal, the sinus or the sublingual space. An adjacent tooth should only be used as a leverage point if it is itself going to be extracted, if the teeth are closely set in the dentition or if there is no other possible support available. Where there is a closely set tooth row a straight elevator can be inserted into the interdental space between the second and third molars; the convex surface should face towards the second molar. The wisdom tooth is then moved upwards and in a distal direction by rotation of the elevator. By deep insertion of the elevator, pressure is transferred on to the alveolar ridge, so that the risk of damaging a tooth is reduced. The applied force is increased by different amounts for individual elevators. It can be raised from 2- to 5-fold. Inclined teeth can also, to a lesser extent, be extracted by this procedure, if the exposure of the tooth is greatly extended mesially or distally.

The final extraction from the socket is achieved by means of special wisdom tooth forceps for upper and lower jaws (**73**), which are used from the front and prevent unnecessary stretching of the soft tissues of the cheek which would arise from lateral insertion.

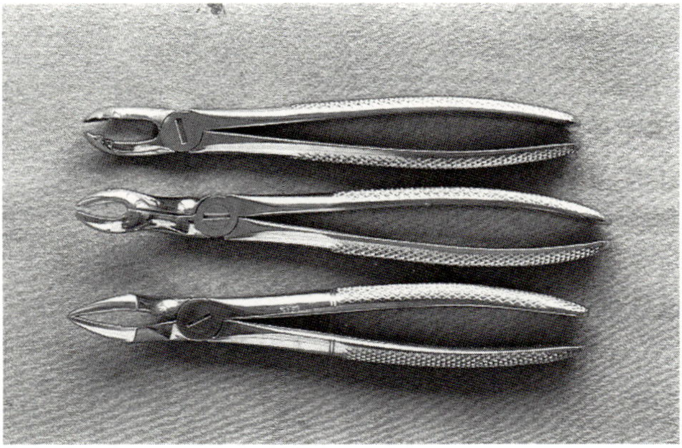

73 Lower jaw forceps, upper jaw forceps and bayonet forceps.

Inclined or horizontal retention

These types of retention necessitate a more extensive exposure of the crown, and in addition the removal of bony tissue distal to the tooth in the case of mesioangular retention and mesial to the tooth in the case of distoangular retention. One should decide about *sectioning* of the tooth soon after exposure of the crown, since the extraction in this way is achieved most easily without further loss of bone. Additional advantages are reduced time of surgery and as a result reduced post-operative wound oedema and reduced danger of damage to adjacent teeth, jaw and inferior alveolar nerve. The sectioning can be carried out either vertically or horizontally with respect to the axis of the tooth (**74, 75**). The

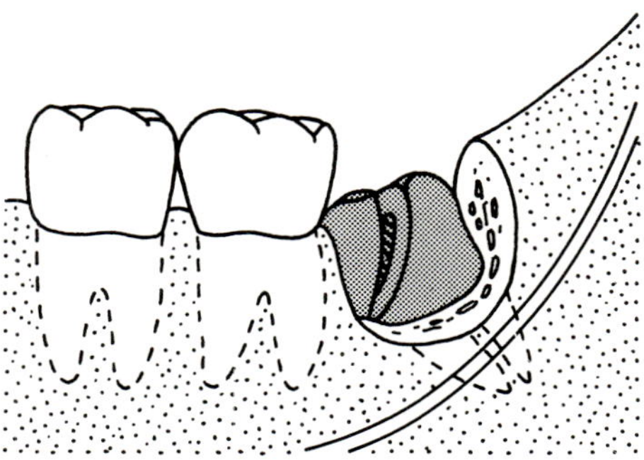

74 Sectioning of an inclined wisdom tooth in the mesioangular position.

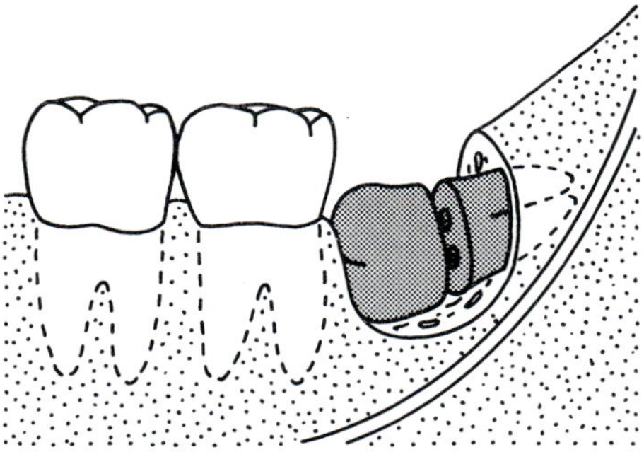

75 Sectioning of a horizontally impacted tooth (mesioangular) at the cemento–enamel junction.

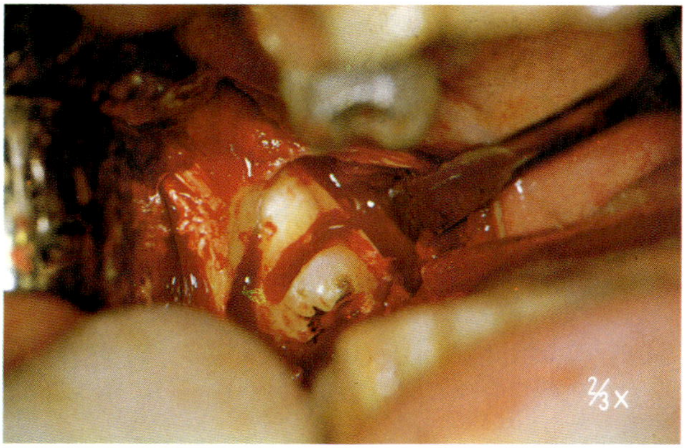

76 Situation following sectioning of a horizontally impacted wisdom tooth.

simplest method is with a Lindemann bur in the region of the cemento-enamel junction; in this case, complete sectioning is unnecessary. The crown can be detached from the root by the insertion and corresponding rotation of a straight elevator (**70, 76**) into a sufficiently deep fissure (ca. 30–40% of the diameter of the root). The extraction of the separate fragments is generally achieved without difficulty, the coronal portion being luxated in the cranial direction and the radicular portion being luxated first in the mesial direction and then in the cranial direction, if it is in the mesioangular position. In the case of inclined teeth in the mesioangular position, division vertical to the tooth axis is carried out if it cannot be extracted despite extensive exposure.

4.5.3 Osteotomy in the upper jaw

Wisdom teeth impacted in the upper jaw are generally simple to extract, as the predominantly spongy bone structure makes extensive osteotomy superfluous. Only in rare cases, where the teeth are extremely displaced, the roots abnormal or the tooth deformed, do significant problems arise, since the anatomical situation prevents a clear exposure and the proximity of the antrum complicates the procedure. In cases of this sort, a transantral extraction may be advisable (Lindorf, 1977).

The vestibular bone layer, which is often very thin, can be removed from above the crown with Rongeurs, a chisel, a periosteal elevator or a bur. After the preparation of an insertion point, usually medial to the crown, the tooth can be luxated in a caudal or vestibular direction with a straight elevator, purely distal movement being avoided because of the danger of fracturing the tuberosity.

4.5.4 Wound revision and closure

After extraction of the tooth the follicle, which is usually attached to the surrounding soft tissue, is removed with a sharp curette, a scalpel or dissecting scissors (**77**). Complete excision is absolutely

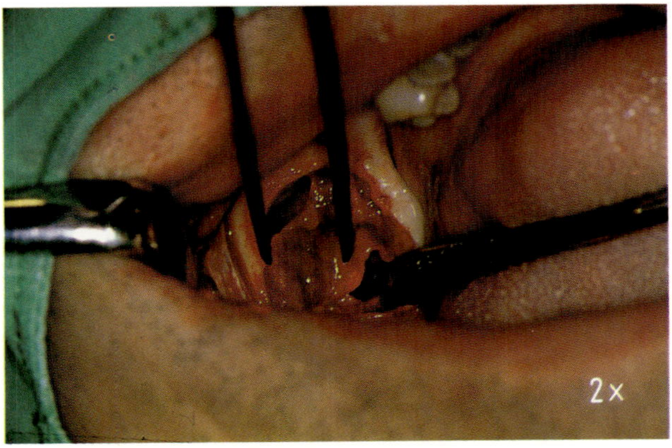

77 Excision of the dental follicle following wisdom tooth extraction.

essential, as cysts may arise from portions of epithelium accidentally left behind (**78**). This is followed by the inspection of the socket. Sharp edges are smoothed down with a round bur or removed with Rongeurs. After bleeding has been stopped, the wound is closed using interrupted sutures for which atraumatic sutures of thread strength 2-0 or 3-0 should be used. We favour braided polyester thread (Mersilene) or resorbable Vicryl sutures, if removal of the sutures is not possible. As a rule, three sutures are sufficient for close approximation of the wound margins (**79**).

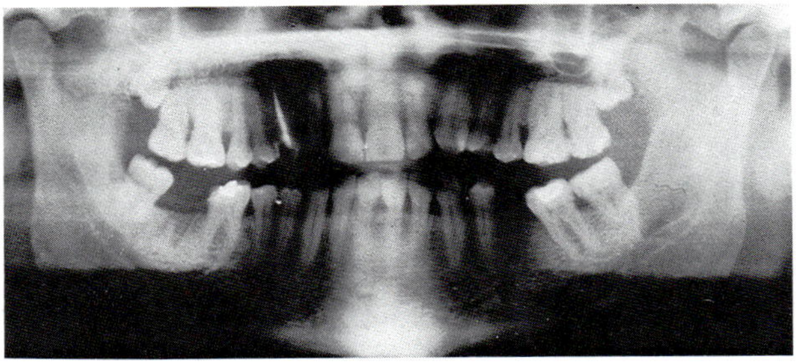

78 Residual cyst in the region of lower left wisdom tooth following surgical extraction of a wisdom tooth in which the follicle was left behind.

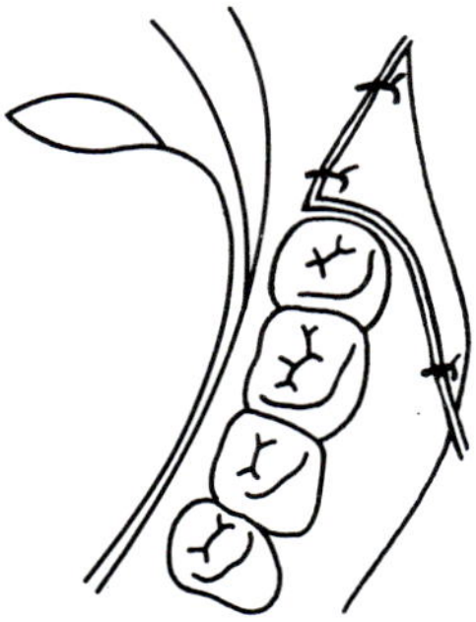

79 Wound closure after surgical extraction of a wisdom tooth.

4.6 Post-operative care

There are three principal methods of after-care:

- primary wound closure (closed after-care),
- drainage (half-open after-care),
- packing (open after-care).

4.6.1 Closed after-care (primary wound closure)

This form of after-care represents the ideal situation. A blood clot forms in the socket and becomes organised into connective tissue and ossified. The requirements for primary healing are a sufficient blood supply, avoidance of trauma and prevention of infection. This after-care is therefore advocated if no infection was present before surgery, if extraction was possible without extensive osteotomy and the general condition of the patient is such that no complications are expected. While this procedure is nearly always possible in the upper jaw – with very few exceptions (less than 1%) – closed after-care can only be undertaken in about one quarter of cases following osteotomy in the lower jaw. The reason for this is the relatively high proportion of therapeutic indications due to infections.

Following wound closure, a bite swab is applied for about 30 minutes. Sutures are removed after 7–10 days. Medication is superfluous in these cases. The use of ice packs is positively beneficial, leading to a significant reduction of wound oedema.

4.6.2 Half-open after-care (drainage)

Where there is extensive infection or danger of infection due to systemic disorders, or following complicated tooth extraction, the socket should be drained for a period of two days after wound closure. A gauze strip is inserted in the vestibular side of the incision by means of a Luniatschek pack applicator (**80**). The strip must only be inserted superficially into the bony cavity, otherwise a stable clot cannot form. The gauze strip merely acts as a means of keeping the incision open and affording an exit for the exudate which is formed. We favour this procedure following extraction of lower wisdom teeth. Drainage from the distal arm of

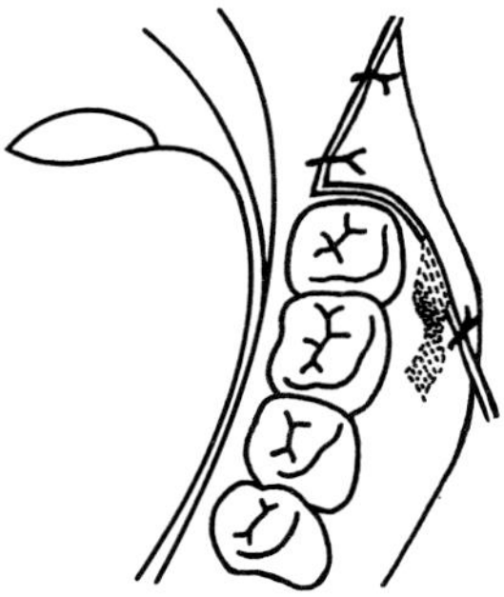

80 Drainage by means of a gauze strip in the mesial arm of the angled incision.

the incision, as sometimes recommended, is less suitable, since it is not at the deepest point, and removal or changing of the dressing causes trouble if there is post-operative stiffness of the jaw. Also, more rapid attachment of the edges of the wound to the bony support is to be expected at the mesial edge of the incision.

On the second post-operative day, the patient is recalled and the strips removed if the wound is healing without complications. Where there is very pronounced oedema of the wound and associated pain, the strips are changed and this must be repeated at regular intervals, depending on the course of healing, until the complications have subsided. In these cases, soaking the strips in chlorophenol–camphor–menthol or ED84 is recommended, as these have analgesic as well as antiseptic properties. If it has to be left for longer, iodoform gauze can also be used (beware of iodine allergies).

In our studies, the average time for which the gauze strip treatment was necessary was 5.4 days. In the 12–40 year age group this is shortened to 5.0 days and in the 41–80 year age group it is lengthened to 8.5 days. While treatment of young patients is completed within one week in 82% of cases, this decreases to 61% in the over-40 age group. In 32.4% of the patients, the drainage strip can be removed after only two days.

4.6.3 Open after-care (packing)

Open treatment following surgical tooth extraction is only rarely indicated (0.3% in our practice). This can be the case in combined therapy, if there is osteomyelitis, an infected cyst or suspected tumour. Packing results in secondary healing, which

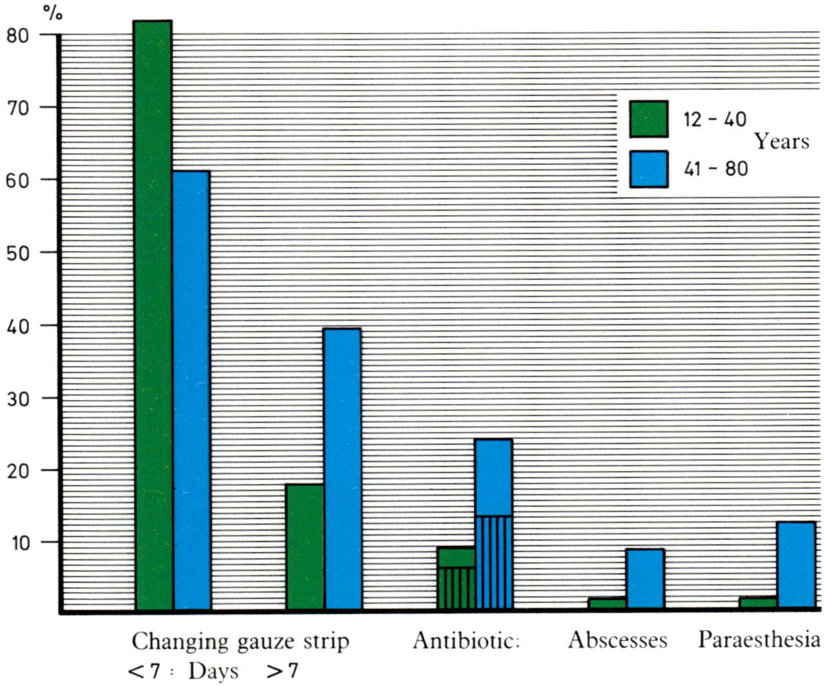

81 Age dependent duration of gauze strip treatment (hatched = longer than 7 days), post-operative abscesses and temporary disturbances of sensation in the area supplied by the inferior alveolar nerve following extraction of lower wisdom teeth.

often necessitates lengthy treatment. The socket must be packed using iodoform dressings at weekly intervals until epithelialisation has taken place. Finally a zinc oxide/eugenol dressing is applied when the complications have subsided. This can be left until it is spontaneously lost through extensive regeneration of the socket. A final check is necessary in every case. Frequently, a deep pocket is left in the bone as a result of this type of treatment and can become the starting point for later complications of an inflammatory nature.

4.6.4 Post-operative Medications

Analgesics

It is usually necessary to prescribe an analgesic following surgery. Among the vast number of preparations mild action analgesics of the antipyretic group, which in addition to the analgesic action possess anti-inflammatory and antipyretic properties, are indicated.

Among the three most important groups – salicylates, p-amino phenols and pyrazolones – a suitable preparation, taking into account the side-effects, should be prescribed or given.

Compound preparations with the addition of codeine, caffeine or barbiturates should only be prescribed in exceptional circumstances where there are good reasons.

Possible antagonistic action with other drugs must be given careful consideration. Thus, patients on *coumarin* must not take salicylates and pyrazolones as the anticoagulant effect of the former can be enhanced, leading to an increased risk of post-operative bleeding (Musch and Gugler, 1981).

Pharmacodynamic interactions can also occur in *diabetics* who are already being treated with oral antidiabetic drugs or insulin. If salicylate (aspirin) is given at the same time, the decrease in blood sugar can be enhanced to the point where hypoglycaemic shock occurs.

In addition, it is necessary to notify patients concerning their *impaired ability to drive,* especially when prescribing narcotic compound analgesics.

Antibiotics

The prophylactic and therapeutic indications for antibiotics are quite different. While therapeutic application must be considered with respect to pre- and post-operative infections, prophylactic use is generally only necessary for inflammation-free tooth extraction when certain systemic disorders are present. With these *problem patients,* in each individual case the possibility of treating them in the practice rather than admitting them to a hospital should be discussed, after consulting their general medical practitioner or consultant.

Where *resistance* is *lowered*, e.g. by cortisone or cytotoxic therapy, radiotherapy, haematological disorders or a severely impaired state of health, prophylactic antibiotic treatment is generally essential; its application must also be considered where there are deleterious effects of infection and a high risk of local infection.

Among the multitude of preparations, penicillin is the first choice for the potential sensitivity spectrum in the oral cavity. Other preparations should only be chosen if there is a known allergy to penicillin and corresponding resistance.

It is particularly important to make sure that the dosage is sufficiently high and that the medication is taken regularly and for a sufficiently long time (see Table 6). In our own investigation, 8.7% of patients aged between 12 and 40 years received an antibiotic. Of these, 2.6% had to take the medication for longer than one week (**81**).

The proportion was significantly higher (23.9%) in the over-40-year-old patients. The proportion of patients who had to be treated with antibiotics for more than one week rose correspondingly (13%).

4.7 Post-operative measures

Oral and written instructions to the patient concerning the procedure following surgery are advisable. They should contain the following information:

Notice concerning restricted driving ability

On the day of the operation, the patient should not drive a vehicle himself. Reaction time may also be slow on the following day if large doses of analgesics with various additives are taken (bear self-medication in mind). In particular the reaction time may well be reduced by the following factors:

- self-medication,
- pain,
- anxiety,
- premedication,
- local anaesthesia,
- surgery,
- post-operative medication.

Local measures

The bite swab can be removed after 30 minutes. On the day of the operation, do not rinse the mouth. On the first post-operative day, the mouth can be washed with lukewarm water, camomile or hydrogen peroxide and on the third post-operative day, careful brushing of the teeth can be started. As a further local measure, ice packs have shown to be excellent for reducing wound oedema.

The patient must be emphatically warned against using warm mouthwashes. Advice about possible bleeding is also recommended; this can be stopped to a certain extent with pressure using a rolled up handkerchief or, with extensive bleeding, another visit to the clinic may be necessary.

Food intake

Eating should not be attempted until the anaesthetic has completely worn off, because of the danger of trauma. On the first three post-operative days, the patient should take only liquid or mashed food. On the day of the operation, the consumption of coffee, alcohol or nicotine is forbidden as it leads to a rise in blood pressure and hence to increased danger of bleeding and infection.

A leaflet should contain information about the analgesic prescribed, the date of the next appointment and in addition a telephone number where the patient can receive information in case of uncertainty.

The following leaflet has proved useful in large oral surgery clinics:

Leaflet concerning the procedure after surgical operation

1. Since driving ability is restricted you should, if possible, not drive a vehicle yourself on the day of the operation. There will be a considerable impairment, especially in the first two hours after the operation.
2. The swelling of the cheeks can be reduced by cooling the cheek on the side where the operation was performed (with ice packs, or plastic bags or hot-water bottles containing ice cubes). *no heat!!!*
3. The bite swab should be removed after thirty minutes.
4. On the day of the operation, no coffee, no alcohol, no nicotine!
5. Do not eat until the anaesthetic has worn off. In the first two to three days, take only liquid or pulped or mashed food.
6. Do not rinse on the first day; on the next day wash mouth with lukewarm water, camomile tea or hydrogen peroxide (one tablespoon of the 3% solution in a glass of water). From the third day, careful brushing of the teeth and more extensive oral hygiene.
7. Minor bleeding can be stopped by applying pressure with a rolled-up handkerchief. If there is more serious bleeding, the clinic must be visited.
8. If the wound is painful, take a maximum of____________ tablets/drops of the prescribed medication. The ability to drive is considerably reduced by high doses, especially if alcohol is consumed as well. If the pain persists, visit the clinic before the date of the next appointment.
9. Date of next appointment:____________________
10. Telephone number for information:____________________

5 SURGICAL PROCEDURE IN SPECIAL SITUATIONS

Numerous pathological changes can occur in conjunction with impacted wisdom teeth. Among these, cystic changes are especially important, since they occur relatively frequently.

5.1 Cysts

Arising especially from lower impacted wisdom teeth are follicular cysts, which can develop to a considerable size without showing symptoms and are often discovered by chance during a radiographic examination (**82, 83**). In every case they must be operated on and the offending wisdom tooth extracted. The appropriate procedure is *cystectomy* (Partsch II): the cyst capsule is removed *in toto* and examined histopathologically. Keratocysts, ameloblastomas (Machtens *et al.*, 1972) and cystic carcinomas can only be diagnosed for certain in this way and treated

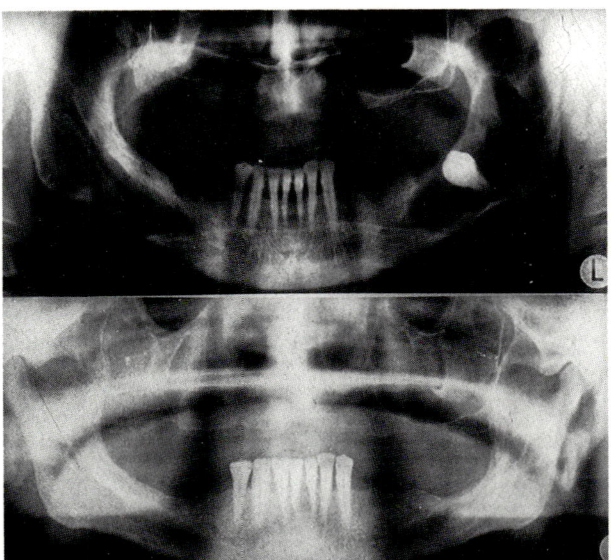

82 Follicular cyst arising from lower left wisdom tooth (above). Bone regeneration 12 months after cystectomy and closed after-care (stabilisation of the blood clot after Schulte).

appropriately. A differential diagnosis must be made in the case of cystic processes, especially in the region of the angle of the jaw, and a great variety of other disorders (**84–86**).

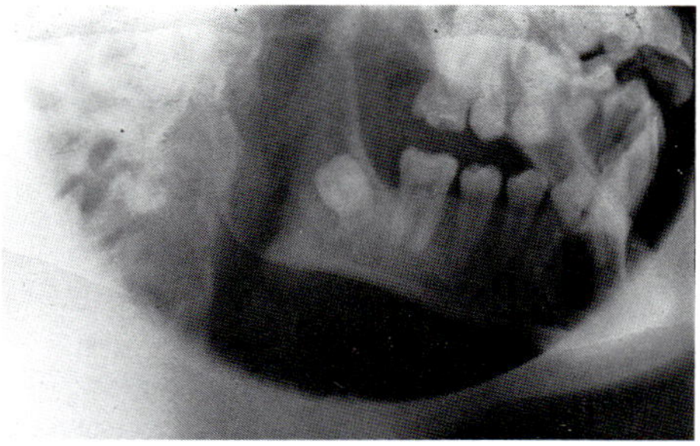

83 Follicular cyst arising from lower right wisdom tooth.

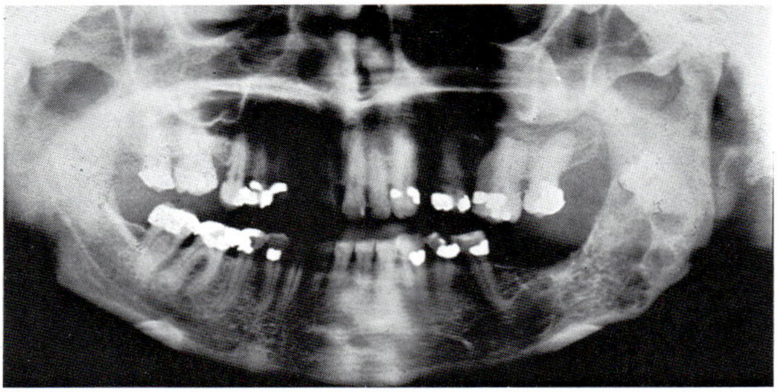

84 Lower left wisdom tooth displaced cranially by solid-cystic ameloblastoma.

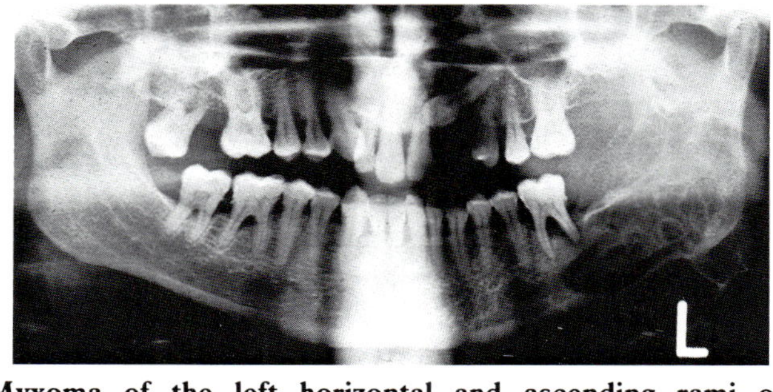

85 Myxoma of the left horizontal and ascending rami of the mandible.

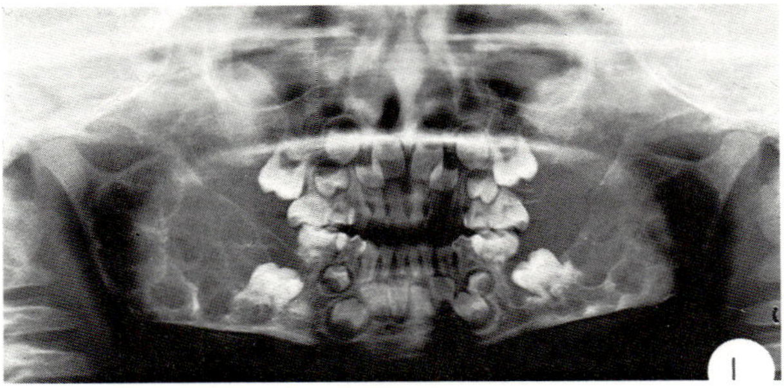

86 Multilocular cystic radiolucency in a 5-year-old boy with cherubism.

Following cystectomy, the cavity in the bone can be treated by open or closed after-care. *Closed* after-care is preferred if there is no infection and the cavity has an extensive bony margin. The size of the cavity plays only a subordinate role in this decision: In cavities over 2 cm in diameter, however, stabilisation of the blood clot by means of Schulte packing (Schulte, 1960) or some other sort of cavity packing (e.g. collagen, Gelastypt M, autologous bone) must be undertaken first of all, as primary healing is not to be expected because of the contraction of the clot and the resultant effusion of serum. The stabilised blood clot requires systemic antibiotic therapy for a period of at least fourteen days.

Cystectomy with open after-care is indicated in those cases where massive infections, complications due to tight wound closure, extensive bone damage or general ailments which predispose to infection are present. In addition, the bone cavity can be utilised, as a form of pre-prosthetic surgical measure, as a means of anchoring a complete denture in an edentulous mandible (**87–89**). The bone cavity is dressed at weekly intervals until it is epithelialised and is finally held open by an obturator or a suitably extended prosthesis.

Cystotomy (Partsch I) is carried out in the same way. Marsupialisation of the cyst is indicated if removal of the cyst capsule would result in damage to important anatomical structures, in particular the inferior alveolar nerve. The latter is quite often displaced by the cyst and can be protected while the capsule is shelled out. Only in rare cases (e.g. following extensive infection) is it fused with the cyst wall, making cystectomy difficult to perform without damaging the nerves; the cyst capsule is at least partially left behind. Cystomy can also be

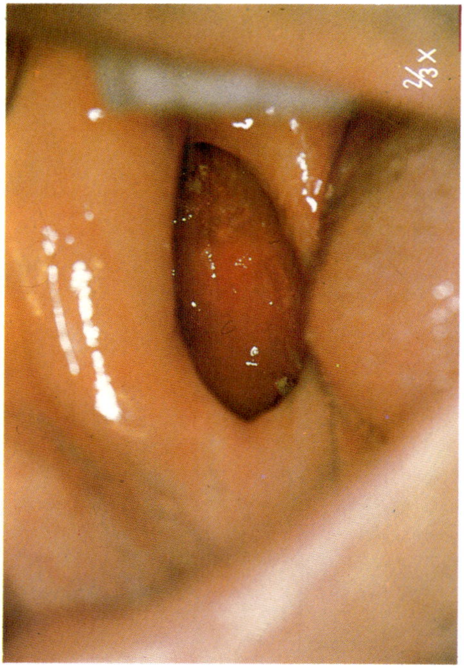

87 Defect in right ascending mandibular ramus following cystectomy and open after-care.

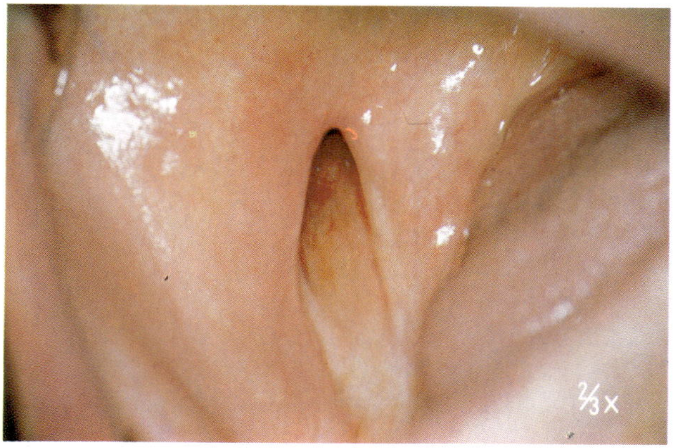

88 Epithelialised residual socket (see **87**) 14 months after operation.

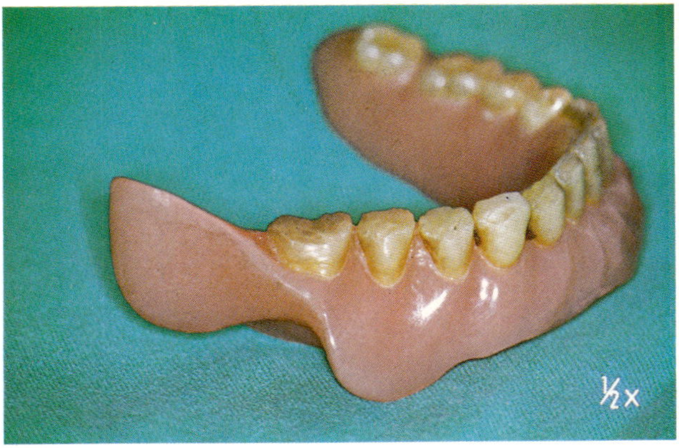

89 Obturator prosthesis (see **87, 88**).

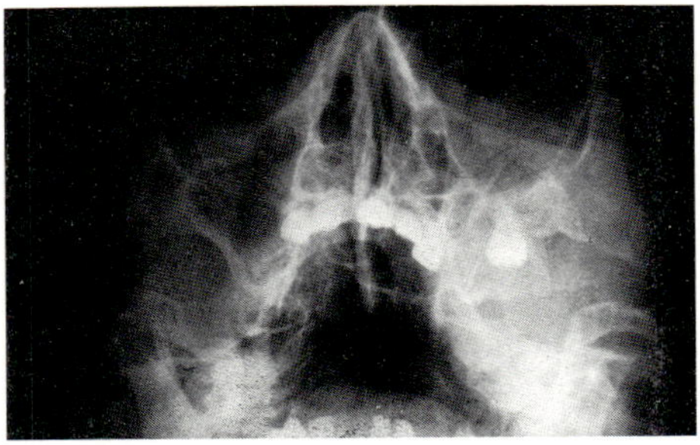

90 Follicular cyst arising from aberrant upper left wisdom tooth.

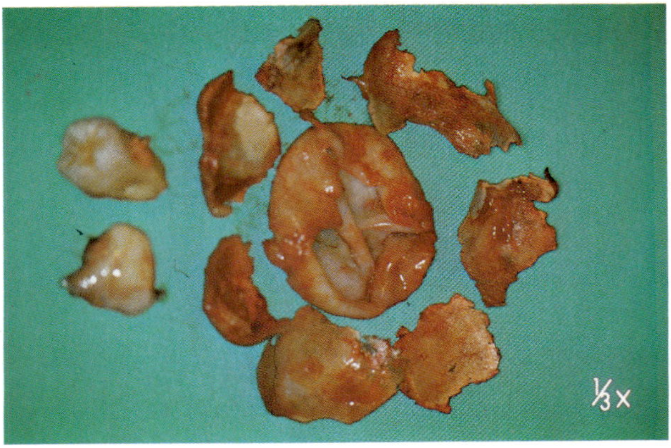

91 Surgical preparation (see **90**). Wisdom tooth, cyst capsule and bone lamellae.

indicated in the case of very large cysts, the complete removal of which can lead to fracture of the mandible through extensive osteotomy. It is possible to perform cystectomy as a secondary operation following bone regeneration. When the cyst epithelium is left in place, open after-care is obligatory, as otherwise there is a high probability of recurrence. However, open after-care in the case of cystic processes in the ascending ramus of the mandible is not without problems, since the masseter and pterygoid muscles can easily bring about premature closure.

Extensive cysts in the upper jaw (**90, 91**) are treated by *antrocystectomy* into the sinus. In this procedure, an additional fenestration of the sinus into the lower nasal passage is necessary to ensure sufficient drainage of the wound exudate. Cysts of this type are sometimes surrounded by a thin layer of bone. This must be removed after shelling out the cyst capsule, since its peripheral portion forms the boundary of a narrow residual sinus. If the bony shell of the cyst is left, an occlusion cyst can arise from the residual sinus if communication with the natural bone or with the artificially produced window has not been established. This operation should be left to specialists in oro-maxillo-facial surgery.

5.2 Fractures

The angle of the jaw is a site predisposed for fractures, on account of the local direction of the bone trabeculae and the presence of impacted wisdom teeth. About 8% of all jaw fractures develop in the region of the angle of the jaw through the socket of an impacted wisdom tooth (Schilli, 1980). The necessity for surgical extraction of the tooth has already been discussed in Section 3.1.5. There is danger of a fracture line osteomyelitis, since communication with the bacteria-laden oral cavity must always be taken into account. The operation is carried out under antibiotic coverage. Luxation must be performed with care in order to avoid dislocation of the jaw fragments. If dislocation has already occurred, the fragments can be wired together during the operation, following suitable reduction (**92**). *Drainage* of the wound cavity is carried out from the vestibular aspect of the incision, as the necessary splinting and immobilisation by means of intermaxillary wiring make after-care difficult. This therapy should be undertaken by suitably experienced specialists. Alternatively, other methods of reduction must be considered in these cases.

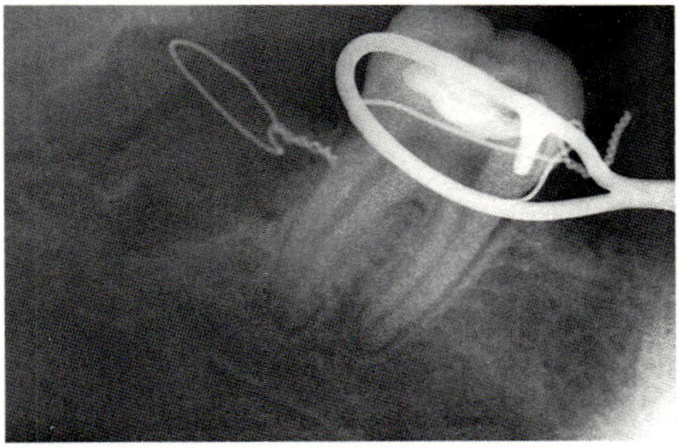

92 Wiring of a fracture of the angle of the jaw following wisdom tooth extraction.

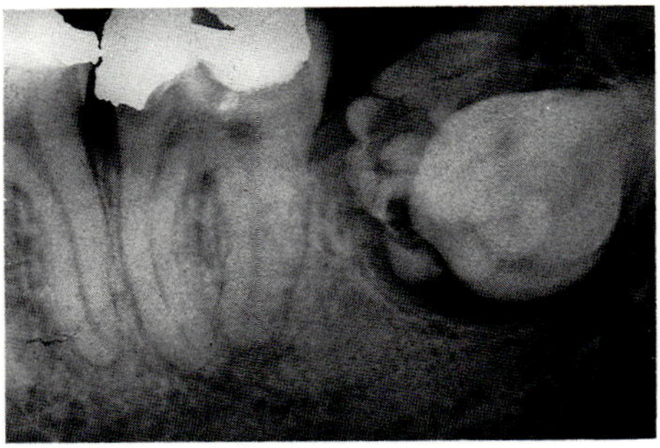

93 Odontoma associated with impacted lower left wisdom tooth.

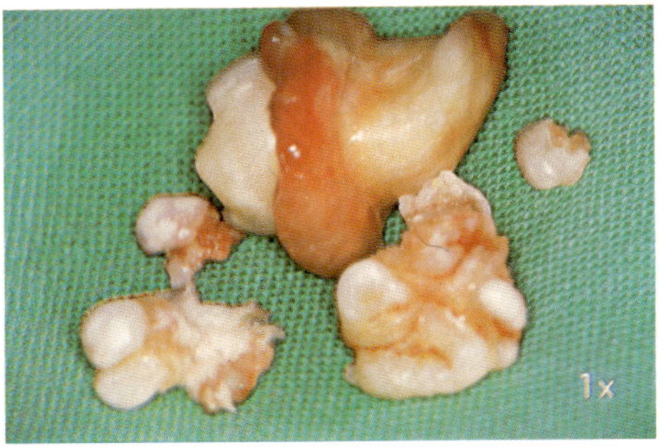

94 Surgical specimen (see **93**).

5.3 Tumours

5.3.1 Benign tumours

Benign tumours of all oral tissues can occur in conjunction with impacted wisdom teeth. Their removal must be carried out in the healthy patient and can be combined with the tooth extraction (**93–96**). Post-operatively every tumour must be examined histopathologically.

Particular attention must be paid to the relatively rare haemangioma of the jaw bone because during tooth extraction massive, uncontrollable haemorrhages can occur. After repositioning of the tooth and suitable compression the patient should be admitted to a hospital without delay.

5.3.2 Semi-malignant tumours

Ameloblastomas occur predominantly in the region of the angle of the jaw. They can be divided into cystic, solid and solid-cystic types. The cystic types frequently show a multi-loculated structure on radiographs (see **49**). Their invasive growth makes a full-scale surgical operation essential; its extent depends on the spread of the tumour. In every case treatment of the patient in a hospital is necessary.

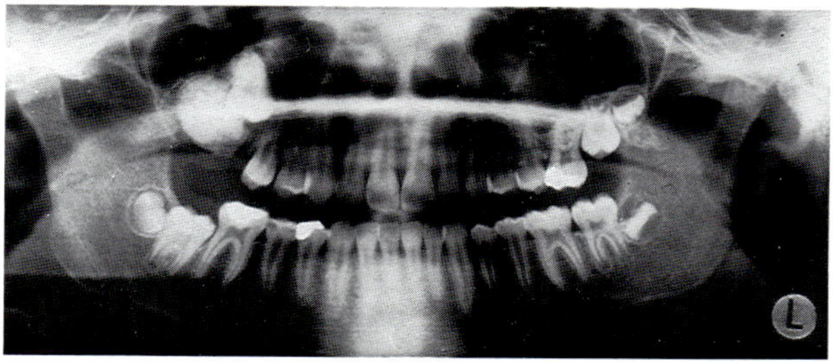

95 Complex odontoma in the region of the cheek teeth in the right upper jaw.

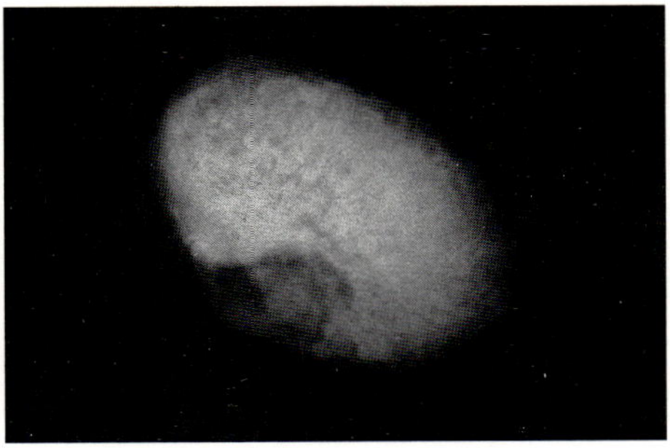

96 Radiograph of excised tumour (see **95**).

5.3.3 Malignant tumours

If wisdom teeth are associated with ulceration of the mucosa or with leucoplastic changes, a malignant tumour must be suspected until proven otherwise by the results of a histopathological examination. This also holds for all radiologically detected osteolytic processes, especially if they show diffuse margins. The inner angle of the jaw is a preferred site for oral carcinoma. These carcinomas have a relatively poor prognosis and can only be treated successfully if diagnosed early. Immediate transfer to a suitable specialist is therefore essential if there is the slightest suspicion.

5.4 Extra-oral tooth extraction

In rare cases the extraction of displaced wisdom teeth in the lower jaw may have to be carried out extra-orally. This method should be chosen if inflammatory processes have led to formation of a fistula – as with chronic granulating periodontitis described by Partsch (**97**). The excision of the fistula can be combined with the extraction of the wisdom tooth. The possibility of damage to the inferior alveolar nerve in the case of teeth located on the base of the mandible or on the buccal aspect is reduced by using the extra-oral route (**98, 99**). Extra-oral wisdom tooth extraction is also possible during the surgical treatment of mandibular fractures; in every case it must be carried out under sterile conditions in a specialised clinic.

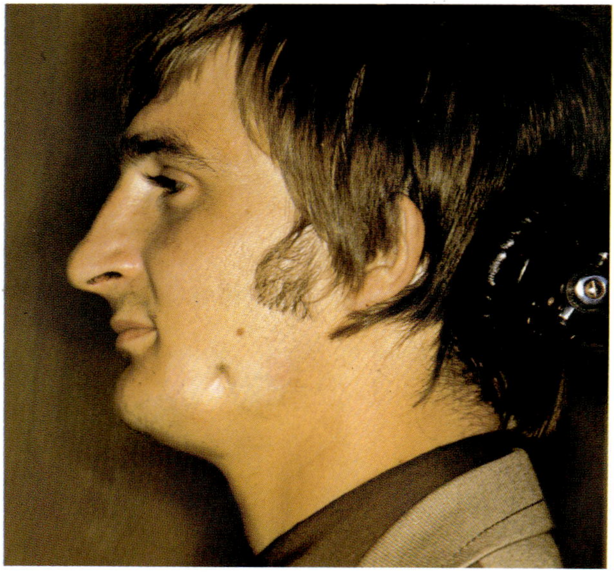

97 Chronic granulating periodontitis as described by Partsch in a case of periapical osteitis of lower left wisdom tooth. Persistent fistula following extraction of the tooth.

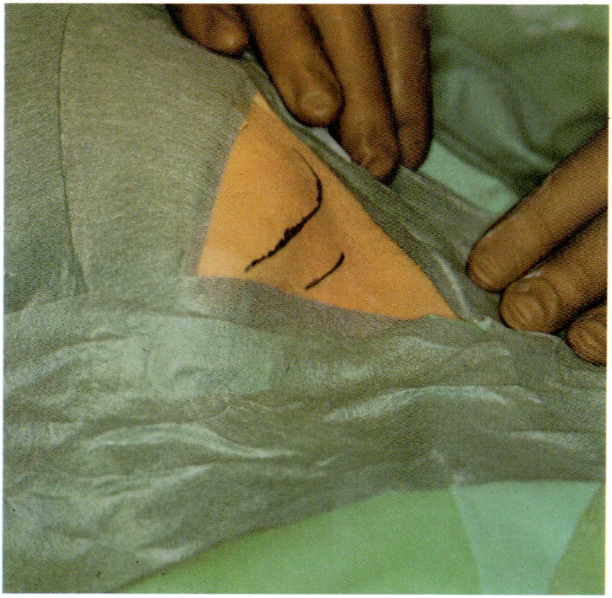

98 Site for extraction of a deep displaced lower left wisdom tooth. Marking of the margin of the lower jaw and the submandibular incision site.

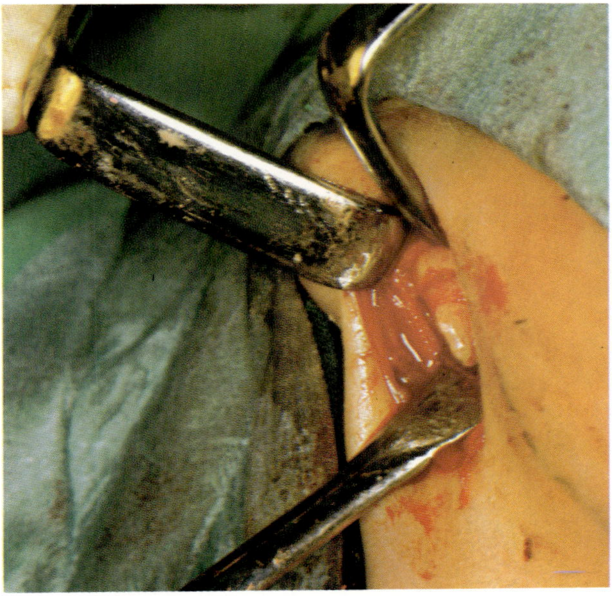

99 Surgical site with exposure of the tooth crown.

5.5 Transantral tooth extraction

Aberrant wisdom teeth in the upper jaw which are located in the maxillary sinus or its walls require transantral extraction. These displaced teeth occur relatively frequently in conjunction with

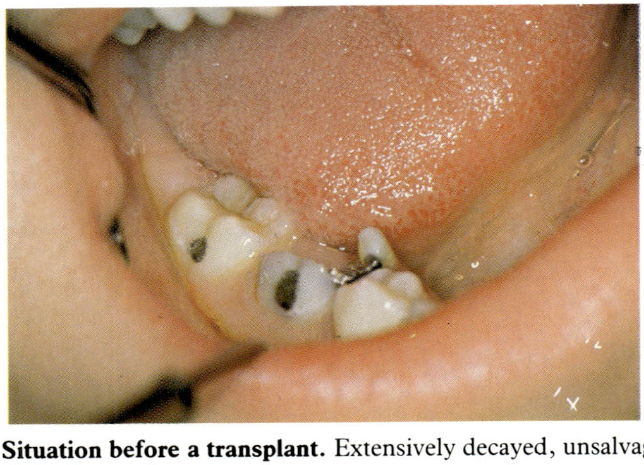

100 Situation before a transplant. Extensively decayed, unsalvageable lower right first molar.

extensive follicular cysts which fill up the entire sinus and can necessitate an extension of the operation due to their expansive nature resulting in displacement of anatomical structures (see **90**).

5.6 Transplantation

Wisdom teeth can be transplanted into the socket of a molar which is not worth saving. Following conservative extraction, in which the root surface must not be damaged, transplantation into the suitably enlarged molar socket is carried out (**100–105**). A one- or two-stage process is currently under discussion. If tooth germs are transplanted into the socket of a molar directly following extraction, blood vessel anastomosis is not always achieved, since the tooth germ rests in point contact on the interradicular septum. Therefore, it is better first to extract the tooth which is not worth keeping and then complete the transplantation after ten days, by which time the socket will have become filled with granulation tissue. After *root development is complete,* some authors recommend transplantation following resection and root canal treatment (**106**), since in the absence of blood vessel anastomosis later treatment of the root is difficult.

In certain cases the allo-autoplastic replantation developed by Kirschner *et al.* (1978) can also be performed. In this procedure the roots of the teeth are shortened by about half, prepared from the apical ends with self-cooling burs and replaced and lengthened with aluminium oxide ceramic posts. With the onset of root resorption the crown of the tooth often remains functional for a longer period.

In addition to autologous tooth or tooth germ transplantation homologous transplantation has been described (Eskici, 1980).

In this treatment, the teeth must be splinted for a 6–8 week period by means of inter-dental fixation.

Opinions differ with respect to the effectiveness of transplants, which often have a limited life span as inflammatory complications and resorptive processes must be expected (**107**). They may be indicated as a temporary measure and treatment attempt in young patients until it is possible to fit a fixed bridge prosthesis. In each case, the indications must be carefully evaluated, bearing in mind alternative forms of treatment.

5.7 Distomolars

Frequently, supernumerary teeth, which are designated disto- or paramolars according to their position, are found in addition to wisdom teeth. In our clinic, these 'nines' are extracted together with wisdom teeth in 0.4% of cases. They occur predominantly in the upper jaw and are mostly rudimentary (**108**). In one case, two distomolars were detected radiographically (**109**). **110** shows these supernumerary tooth rudiments in three quadrants.

The surgical procedure differs from wisdom tooth extraction only in that the exposure must be more extensive; the danger of penetrating the sinus is therefore greater.

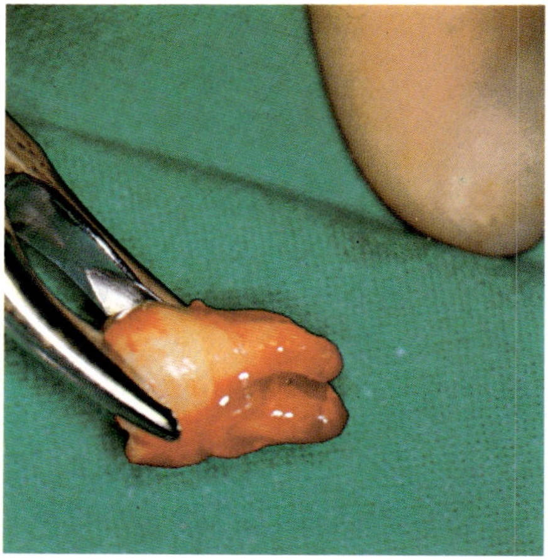

101 **Surgically extracted lower right wisdom tooth with intact periodontal ligament.**

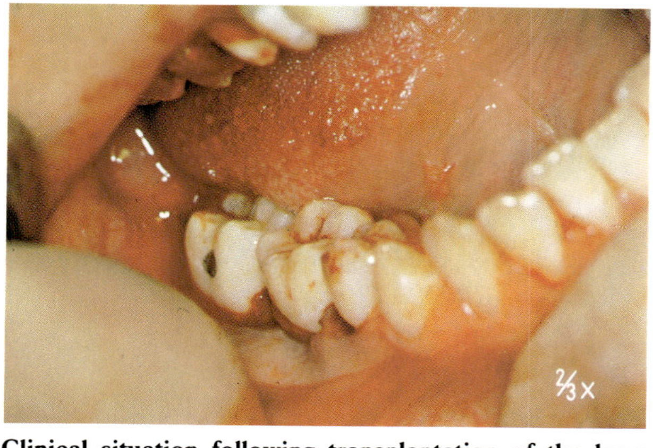

102 **Clinical situation following transplantation of the lower right wisdom tooth in the socket of the ipsilateral first molar.**

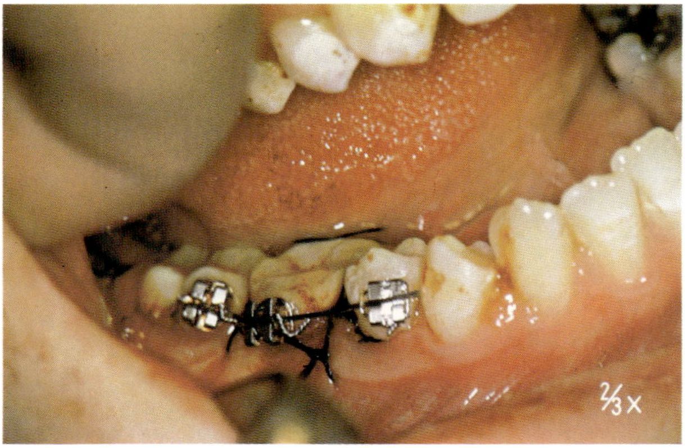

103 Situation following splinting of the transplanted lower right wisdom tooth.

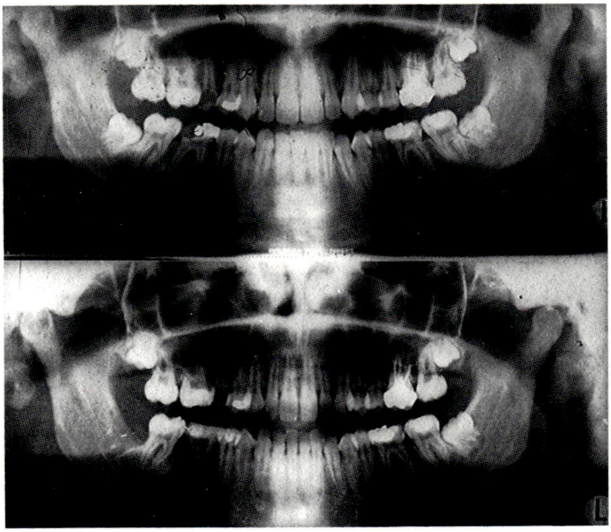

104 Pre- and post-operative radiographs.

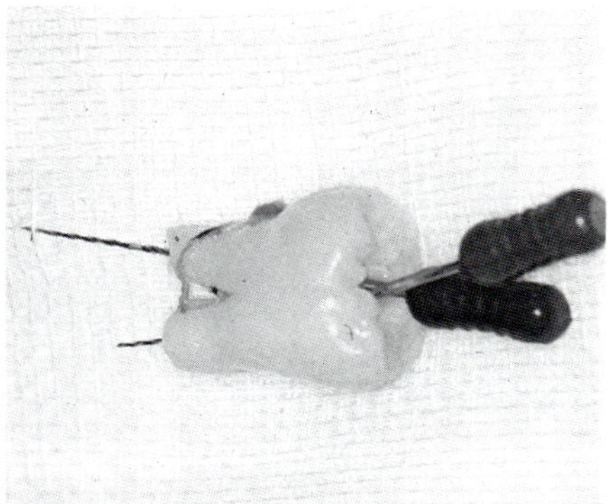

105 Situation following extirpation of the pulp and apicectomy of a wisdom tooth before transplantation.

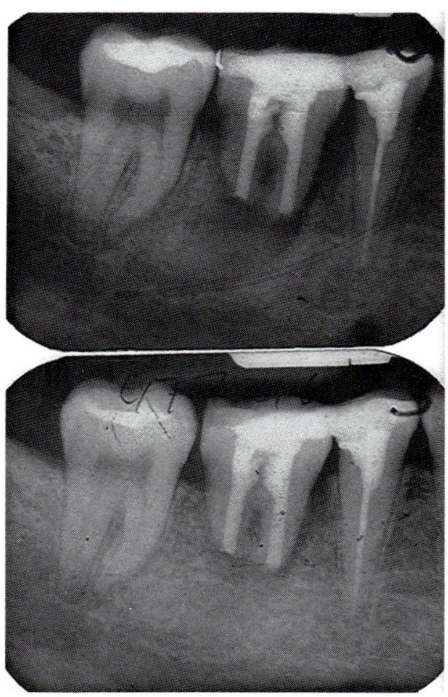

106 Situation following transplantation of a root canal treated lower right wisdom tooth. Immediately after the operation (above) and 2 years post-operatively (below).

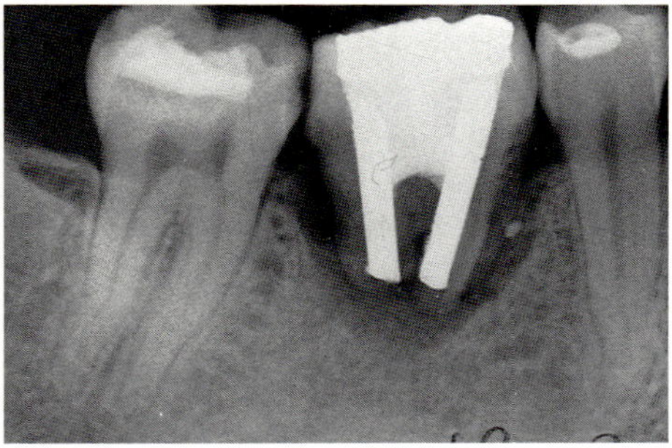

107 Extensive breakdown of bone and inflammatory complications 12 months after a transplant.

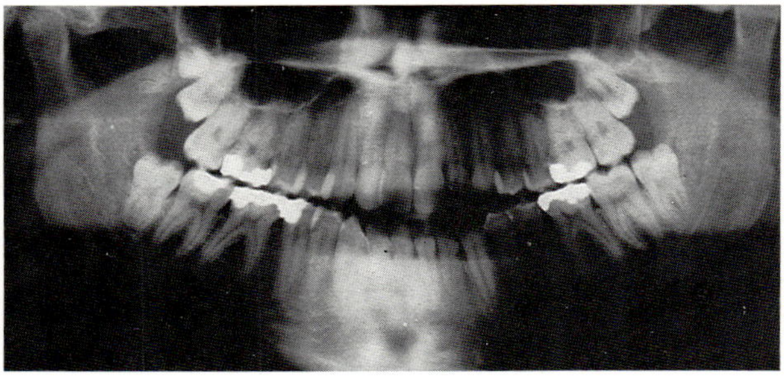

108 Distomolar in right upper jaw.

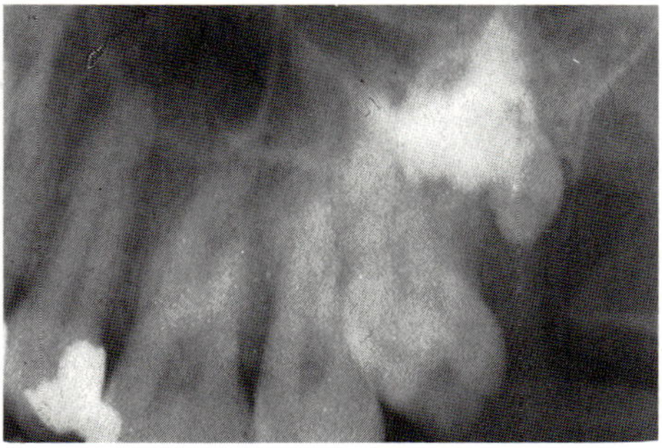

109 Two distomolars in left upper jaw.

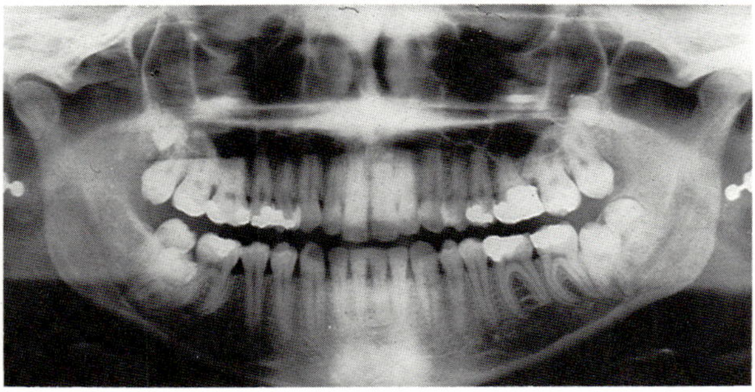

110 Distomolars in both upper quadrants and in the lower left quadrant.

6 COMPLICATIONS

6.1 Complications during surgery

6.1.1 Dental complications

Tooth fractures and displacements

Fracture of the crown or root is the most common complication of tooth extraction. Since a relatively high percentage of wisdom teeth show abnormalities of the roots (**111, 112**), root fracture occurs more frequently. The danger of small root fragments remaining in the jaw, the removal of which would present considerable problems, can be reduced by extensive exposure and sectioning of the tooth. Fragments must be removed with great care, following excision from the bone, using small forceps in order to prevent luxation into the inferior dental canal, the maxillary sinus or the infratemporal space. If the lingual bony plate is damaged, displacement into the sublingual or parapharyngeal space is also possible and this causes problems because of the large number of nerves and blood vessels; the lingual nerve in particular is placed in jeopardy.

The risk of removing small root fragments of vital wisdom teeth must be weighed against the possible complications which may ensue from leaving them in each individual case. If removal is decided against, the patient must be advised of the situation and made aware of the danger of possible infections.

Special problems occur with teeth showing *hypercementosis*. Without complete exposure as far as the often bulbous thickening of the root apex, extraction is impossible. Similar difficulties occur with older patients, if the teeth are ankylosed with the surrounding bone. A periodontal space is no longer present if the ligament has calcified and the tooth can be separated from the bone only with great difficulty. In these cases, intra-operative radiographs may be necessary to clarify the situation. Similar problems also occur with teeth which have been non-vital for a long time. They crack like glass while being extracted and must be removed in fragments.

Excessive use of force when inserting elevators should be

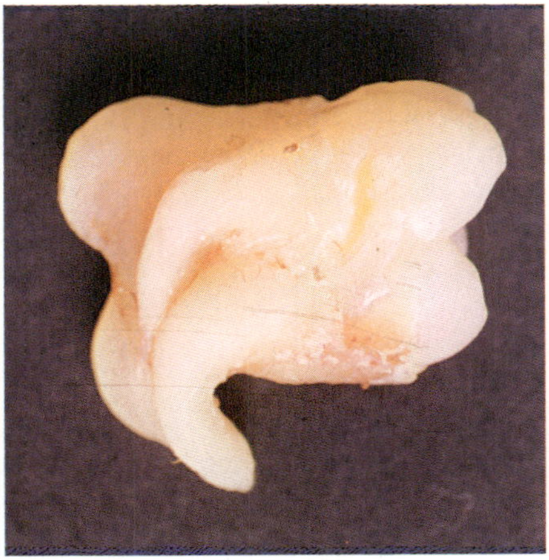

111 Distally recurved roots of a lower wisdom tooth.

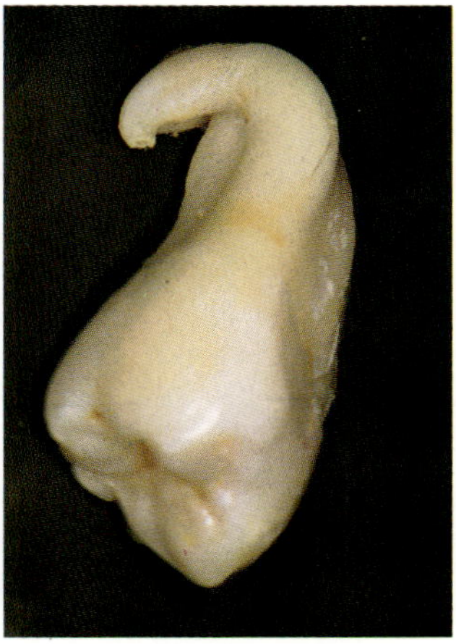

112 Extreme curvature of the roots of an upper wisdom tooth.

avoided, since damage to neighbouring teeth and surrounding bone may occur. Tooth damage of this sort is often a sure sign of the improper use of elevators.

The use of forceps without the necessary support may lead to damage of the antagonists. Such damage is avoided by correct operative technique.

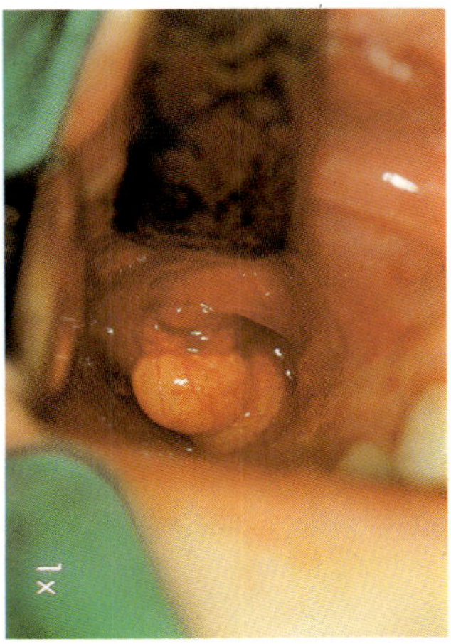

113 Prolapse of buccal pad of fat during extraction of an upper wisdom tooth.

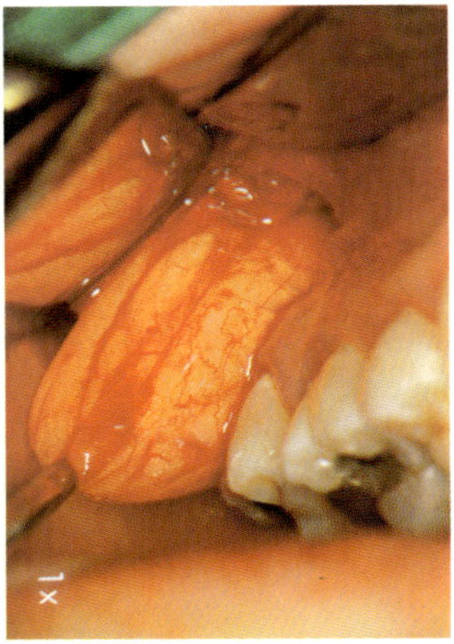

114 Displacement of buccal pad of fat into the oral cavity (see **113**).

Swallowing and aspiration

Teeth are swallowed or aspirated relatively rarely. Swallowing as a rule has no serious consequences. The tooth leaves the body through the digestive tract. A radiograph is necessary only in exceptional circumstances.

Aspiration is an *emergency*. It can lead to respiratory insufficiency as a result of mechanical obstruction or to reflex respiratory failure. The immediate removal of the tooth with the aid of a bronchoscope by an ENT specialist is absolutely essential.

Coughing fits can occur as a result of aspiration. If aspiration is suspected, a radiograph of the lungs should always be taken.

6.1.2 Soft tissue complications

Damage

Soft tissue complications can arise as a result of damage due to incorrect manipulation of retractors. Extreme traction should also be avoided out of consideration for post-operative oedema. If the operation site is sufficiently exposed the retractors can be held in place without the use of force. Extensive damage can result from the bur slipping off into the soft tissue. The instrument must be removed carefully and the wound sutured. Haemorrhage and nerve damage are possible in situations of this sort. Complications can be avoided by suitable support, by careful use of the handpiece and by protecting the soft tissue with a periosteal elevator.

There is a significant correlation between the duration of the operation and post-operative wound oedema. This is due primarily to trauma inflicted on the soft tissues by retractors.

Haemorrhages

Intra-operative haemorrhages occur relatively frequently. They can be divided into arterial, venous or tissue haemorrhages. While bleeding from blood vessels is arrested by clamping, tying off, suturing or coagulation, closure of the wound and subsequent compression by means of a bite swab is indicated for tissue haemorrhage. Only in the case of prolonged bleeding is the socket packed. Denatured cellulose (Tabotamp) has proved the most suitable packing material.

Haemorrhages during extraction of a wisdom tooth can usually be overcome by local measures, if haemorrhagic disorders are not believed to be the cause. The latter are divided into coagulopathies, thrombopathies and vasopathies and ought to be diagnosed pre-operatively by a specialist and treated appropriately. A similar problem exists with iatrogenic clotting deficiency (e.g. coumarin therapy). Severe haemorrhages can result from haemorrhagic bone cysts.

Prolapse of the buccal pad of fat

A further – albeit harmless – complication during extraction of upper wisdom teeth is a prolapse of the buccal pad of fat (**113, 114**). Treatment consists of repositioning and subsequent wound closure.

Emphysema

Emphysema has rarely been described in connection with wisdom tooth extraction. It consists of accumulation of air in the tissues, which can have many causes. According to the investigations of Neuner (1977), the use of the high speed air rotor in osteotomy is the main cause; this was first described by Charlebois (1964) following surgical extraction of wisdom teeth with the aid of the air rotor. Kilpatrick and Yonkers (1958) and Hall (1959) advocate its use, since it shortens the operation time, reduces post-operative swelling and the danger of damage and promotes wound healing. The disadvantages are the possibility of spreading infection, thermal damage to bone and occurrence of air emphysema, which can be attributed to the drive air pressure (up to 4 atm) and the spray air pressure (up to 2 atm).

Increases in *intra-oral pressure* can be mentioned as a further complication during and after wisdom tooth extraction; these can arise as a result of sneezing, snoring, coughing, blowing the nose, playing a wind instrument or from severe physical exertion. Post-operative rinsing with high concentrations of hydrogen peroxide has been suggested as a cause of complications (1 ml of a 30% solution can liberate 100 ml of oxygen). Therefore, only 1% up to a maximum of 3% solutions should be used for wound treatment.

The spread of emphysema follows the line of least resistance of the tissue. It therefore spreads into muscle spaces, blood vessels and nerve channels, the crevices between fasciae and the porous part of the connective tissue within seconds or hours. The swelling can remain confined to one side of the face or can spread to the opposite side or downwards as far as the mediastinum.

The *consistency* of emphysema is spongy and elastic. *Snowball crepitations* can be felt on digital palpation. Patients often complain of pressure pain or a feeling of constriction; a rise in temperature, shivering and sweating are signs of an infection necessitating antibiotic treatment. Therapy consists of treatment of the mental state of the frequently distressed patient – possibly by prescription of sedatives – and physical measures (alternate warm and cold compresses, infra-red radiation, pressure dressings and alcohol or borax poultices).

A feeling of pressure in the thoracic region and difficulty in breathing are signs of *mediastinal emphysema*. In these cases, a thoracic examination is necessary. With increasing impairment of lung, heart and circulatory functions, suprasternal incision and drainage may be required to prevent death.

To prevent facial emphysema arising during or after dental surgical operations, the following points should be observed:

- avoidance of high speed air rotors for osteotomy,
- advising the patient to avoid increasing intra-oral pressure (in particular glass-blowers and players of wind instruments),
- tight wound closure and additional use of tissue adhesives in patients at risk,
- avoidance of high concentrations of hydrogen peroxide in wound treatment.

6.1.3 Nerve complications

Local anaesthesia

Nerve damage can occur as early as during the injection of an anaesthetic. Although this complication is very rare if faultless injection materials and correct injection technique are used, it cannot be avoided with complete certainty. If a shooting pain occurs when the needle is inserted, the position of the needle must always be changed before delivery of the anaesthetic. The danger of direct damage can be practically eliminated by the use of very thin, disposable needles. It is a different matter if the local anaesthetic is injected into the nerve trunk; toxic damage to the nerve, causing loss or restriction of function, is then possible.

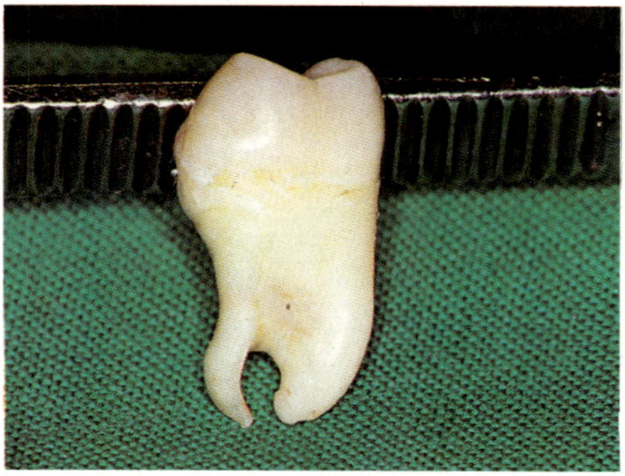

115 Interradicular course of the inferior alveolar nerve.

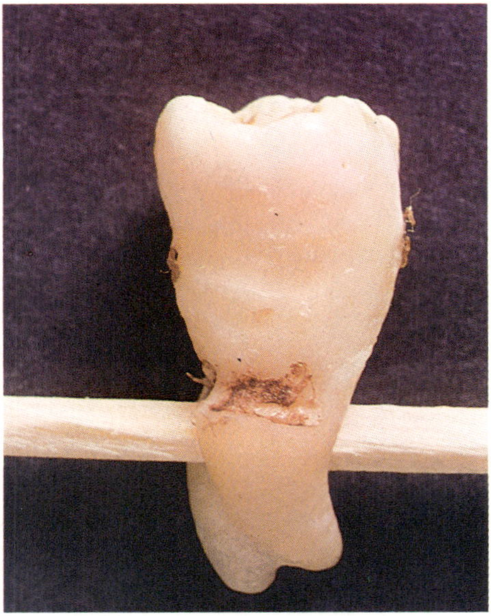

116 Interradicular course of the nerve in an enclosed canal.

The duration of the resulting complete or partial anaesthesia is highly variable and may be associated with unpleasant paraesthesia. In rare cases, the damage is permanent. This is more common in older patients and is particularly disturbing when the lingual nerve is involved.

In addition to loss of sensation in one half of the tongue, disturbances of taste occur, since the nerve carries with it gustatory fibres from the chorda tympani. The prognosis for damage to the lingual nerve is especially poor.

Temporary loss of function may be caused by a *haematoma* which has arisen as a result of damage to a blood vessel during anaesthesia; sensation usually returns within a few days or weeks.

The *therapeutic possibilities* for nerve damage are limited. Medically, if a haematoma is present, drugs can be prescribed to reduce the swelling. The action of neurotropic vitamins (e.g. Neurobione) is not guaranteed. Their prescription certainly helps the relationship between patients and the surgeon, whom they have often lost faith in. Psychological support can therefore be very important. If confidence has been lost, it is advisable to refer the patient to a specialist. The therapeutic possibilities are not much greater here, but the patient can obtain the opinion of a third party and this often restores his confidence in the surgeon. He should in any case be informed that a six-month regeneration time is to be expected.

Surgery

As a rule, nerve damage occurring during the operation is avoidable. The specific anatomical situation in the angle of the jaw and its effect on the incision and surgical procedure have already been discussed. Lingual osteotomy should be restricted to those cases in which the wisdom tooth is displaced lingually. Scrupulous subperiosteal preparation and the protection of the soft tissues with a suitable retractor, spatula or periosteal elevator during osteotomy are important factors in avoiding damage to the lingual nerve.

The situation is more complicated in the case of *deeply displaced wisdom teeth* which are in contact with the inferior alveolar nerve. The nerve can be trapped by a wisdom tooth or in extreme cases may even run interradicularly in an enclosed canal (**115–118**). If this situation has not been detected, the nerve will inevitably be severed on extraction. By proceeding with care one can establish, in cases of this sort, that the tooth is elastically attached during extraction, in spite of extensive mobility. Several authors also consider a sudden pain caused by a pull on the inferior alveolar nerve to be a criterion of tooth–nerve associations of this kind. From our own experience, we must say that this criterion is unreliable. This complication should be suspected if there is radiologically demonstrable superposition of the wisdom tooth and the inferior dental canal – especially if there is a change in

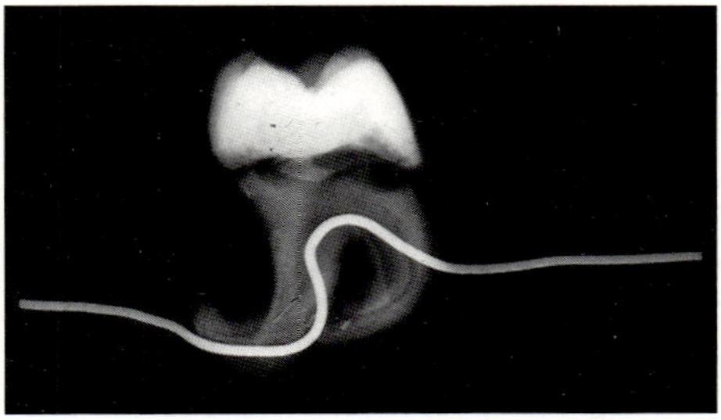

117 Abnormal interradicular nerve route with change of direction (reconstruction using a wire).

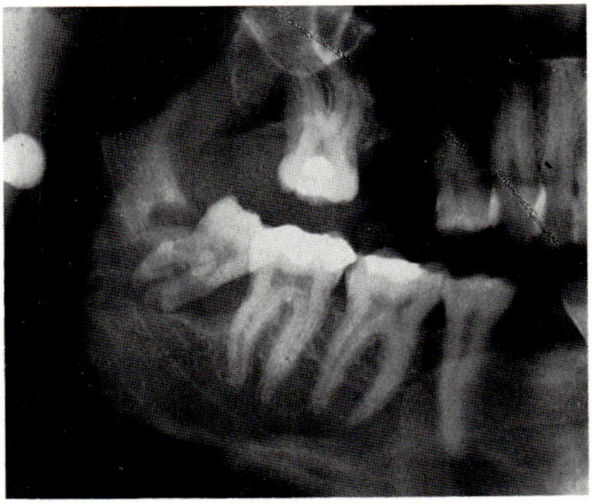

118 Lower right wisdom tooth elastically attached during extraction (nerve running interradicularly).

direction in the course of the canal. A radiograph of suitable dimensions to ensure an adequate survey of the area is required.

If there is simply *contact* between the *root apices* and the *canal* or if, indeed, the latter is opened during extraction of the wisdom tooth, there is generally no danger of damaging or severing the nerve. On the other hand, haemorrhages from the associated, relatively thin-walled veins often occur. These are easily stopped by compression but the canal should not be packed in these cases, as the nerve may be damaged by the pressure.

If extraction using elevators is carried out carelessly, there is the danger of perforating the *roof of the inferior dental canal,* in which case a root fragment may drop into the canal. The resultant haemorrhage complicates subsequent procedure. The root must always be removed, otherwise neuralgiform pain, neuralgia, neuritises or loss of function may occur. The roof of the canal is carefully removed with a round bur until the root is visible and can be extracted. Instruments designed for removing calculus may be helpful for this. Where the inferior alveolar nerve or the lingual nerve is *severed* during extraction of a wisdom tooth, the patient should be referred to a maxillofacial surgery clinic equipped to deal with microsurgical nerve repair and, depending on the diagnosis, give expert advice on primary or secondary nerve reconstruction. The practising dentist, oral surgeon or specialised physician, by referring the patient in this way, covers himself against judicial claims that possible long-term consequences were recognised too late and treated incorrectly (Scheunemann and Hausamen, 1980).

It is impossible to give an unequivocal answer to the question of *surgical nerve reconstruction*. Lingual reconstruction does not succeed in restoring the loss of taste, which is very distressing to the patient. Neither can restoration of sensation following this type of operation be guaranteed (Scheunemann and Hausamen, 1980).

Following extraction of lower wisdom teeth we have observed partial anaesthesia or paraesthesia in 1.5% of cases in the 12–14 year age group. The percentage increases considerably among older patients (12%; see **81**). However, only in one case did a partial loss of sensation of the lower lip last for more than 12 months after the operation (Herz, 1982).

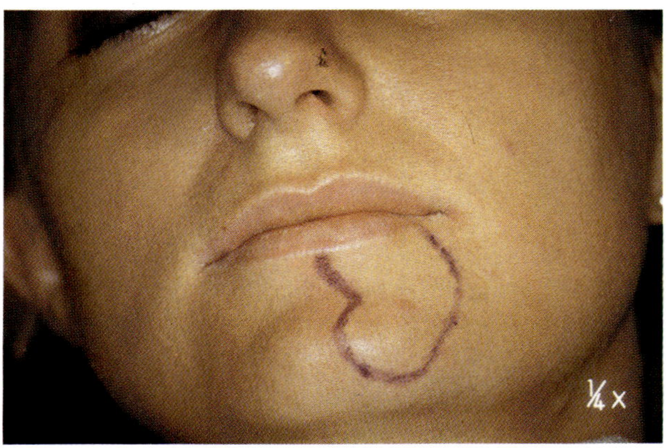

119 Outlining the region of loss of sensation following nerve damage through extraction of a lower left wisdom tooth.

Post-operative oedema and haematomas

Irritation of a nerve with temporary loss of function is also possible as a result of post-operatively occurring oedema or haematomas. The disturbances of sensation disappear along with their cause.

In cases of trauma to the inferior alveolar nerve it may be advisable to estimate the area of reduced sensitivity on the lower lip by means of a sharp probe, to mark it and document it photographically (**119**). In this way, one can visualise the extent of regeneration at a later examination and give the patient some assessment of any progress which has been made. This procedure also has a positive effect on agitated patients. In addition, reduced sensation, paraesthesia or anaesthesia of the Vincent symptom type is an indication of the onset of osteomyelitis.

6.1.4 Bone complications

Haemorrhages

Haemorrhages from vessels in the bone, arising during surgery, can be controlled by coagulation or by compression. In electrocoagulation a probe or claw is inserted into the opening in the bone and coagulation achieved with the electrotome. Closure of blood vessels by compression is carried out with a chisel and light hammer blows, knocking the surrounding bony tissue into the bleeding bone canal. This procedure should be avoided in the vicinity of the mandibular canal, as it may damage the inferior alveolar nerve.

Fracture of the mandible

A fracture during wisdom tooth extraction is a dramatic event. The displaced wisdom tooth results in weakening of the jaw; this is the cause of about 8% of all jaw fractures and about 20% of fractures of the mandible near the angle of the jaw which, together with the condyles, represent the most common site for fracture.

Spontaneous fractures are also observed in this region in cases of massive osteolytic activity or extreme atrophy. *Iatrogenic fractures* occur if, during extraction of an impacted tooth, excessive force is exerted in a mesiodistal direction – exacerbated by the use of unsuitable elevators – without the removal of

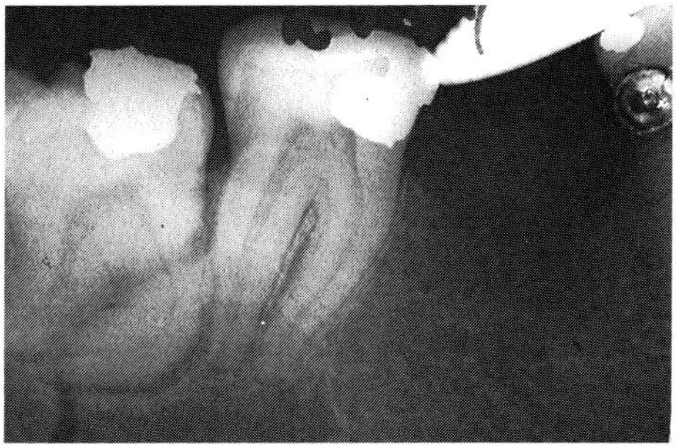

120 Fracture of the mandible following attempt to extract lower right wisdom tooth.

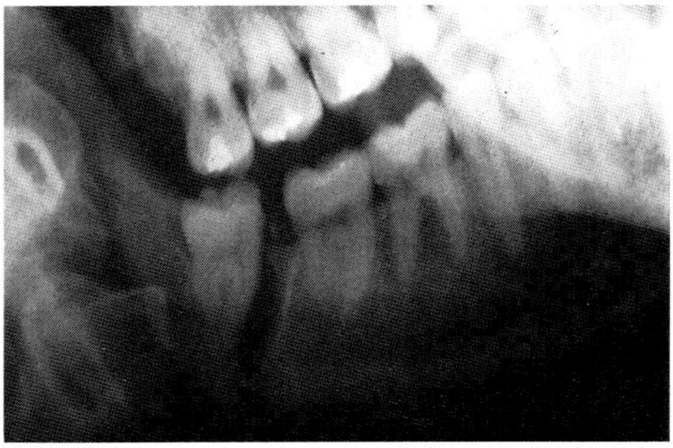

121 Fracture of the mandible following attempt to extract lower right wisdom tooth with interdental insertion of the elevator and distal luxation.

enough bone (**120, 121**). In these cases, the bone in the region where the tooth is to be exposed must be excised. On the other hand, the jaw is weakened by extensive osteotomy. The greater the osteotomy needed to expose the tooth the smaller must be the force applied to luxate and then extract the tooth.

About 1% of jaw fractures are iatrogenic. It has been shown that they occur predominantly in the course of extraction of lower wisdom teeth. However, in relation to the total number of teeth extracted, they must be regarded as decidedly rare. In an evaluation of ten fractures of this type it was noteworthy that in only three cases was the fracture discovered at once and the patient referred for further treatment. In two cases detection was delayed by one week, in four cases by 3–5 weeks and in one case further treatment was not received until 3 months later (Haunfelder and Tetsch, 1972). The danger of fracture is especially great where deep displaced teeth in an atrophied and sclerotic jaw have abnormal roots or are ankylosed. Pathological processes such as cysts, osteomyelitis, tumours and skeletal disorders can enhance the risk considerably. In such cases, prophylactic splinting before the operation is advisable.

It is not always easy to establish that a fracture has occurred. If on overcoming persistent resistance, suspicious sounds and abnormal movements occur this should be an indication for the operator to take radiographs in two planes, since this is the only means by which fractures can be excluded with certainty and dislocations discovered.

On diagnosis of a fracture, the patient must be advised of the situation before appropriate measures are undertaken. In every case further treatment must be carried out by an experienced oral surgeon with specialised knowledge, who has command of the various treatment possibilities of conservative splinting and surgical reduction of fractures and who institutes the appropriate procedure.

Since events of this kind often have forensic consequences, referral to a suitable specialist or hospital is emphatically advised because, apart from the question of responsibility for the fracture, a review of the treatment of the fracture often forms the starting point for legal proceedings.

A jaw fractured during wisdom tooth extraction is regarded as an 'atypical danger' because of its extremely rare incidence and certainly does not need to be included in the general pre-surgical information. However, on consideration of particular cases there may be a responsibility to inform the patient about the possible risk of fracture. This holds for tooth extraction from jaws where there are pathological changes, or from jaws atrophied by old age. The evaluation of a pre-surgical survey radiograph can lead to the discovery of such changes and allows corresponding treatment plan modifications.

Fracture or abscission of the tuberosity

In general, extraction of wisdom teeth from the upper jaw presents no great problem because it is facilitated by the spongy structure of the bone. The direction of luxation is generally distobuccal. For this the crown must be sufficiently exposed or it is possible for the tooth and the tuberosity to be displaced distally together during luxation, leading to fracture (**122, 123**). This danger is particularly great in the case of ankylosed or isolated teeth and abnormal roots. As long as the tuberosity is attached to

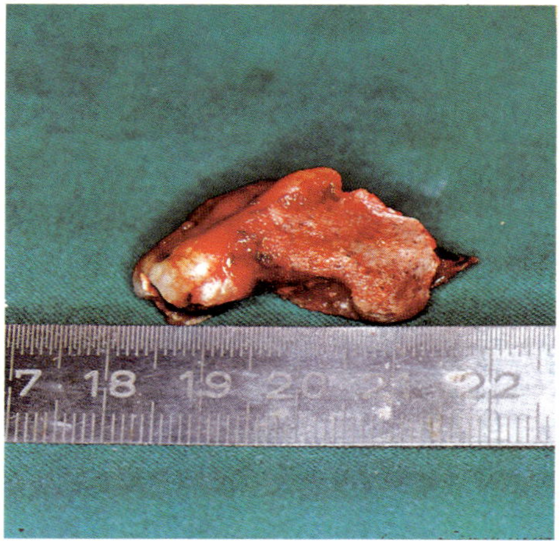

122 Upper right wisdom tooth with the right tuberosity, following abscission of the tuberosity.

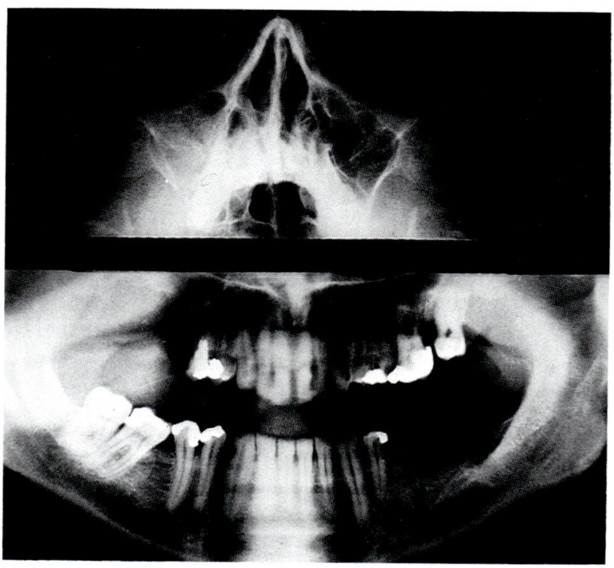

123 Nasal cavity radiograph and orthopantomogram following abscission of the tuberosity.

the mucous membrane by a peduncle and thus supplied by it, it can be replaced after extraction of the tooth and immobilised after union of the mucous membrane by means of a Miniplast plate. Precise wound closure assumes a particular importance since following abscission of the tuberosity the maxillary sinus is wide open and secondary closure in this inaccessible area is difficult.

In the case of *complete removal of the tuberosity* with the tooth a free transplantation is not very promising. In these cases it is

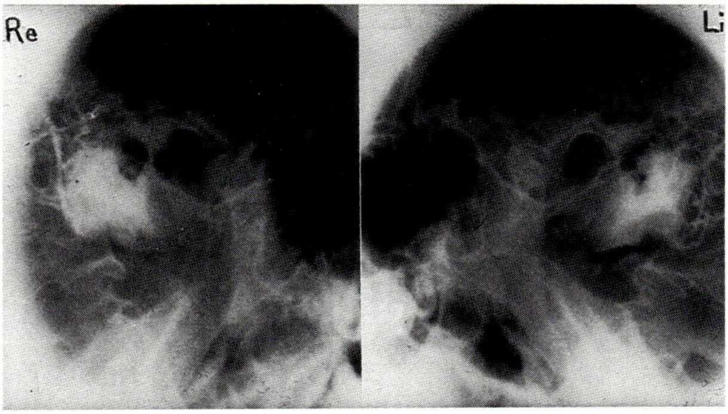

124 Joint radiograph after Schüller (transcranial joint radiographs), showing bilateral fixed joint dislocation.

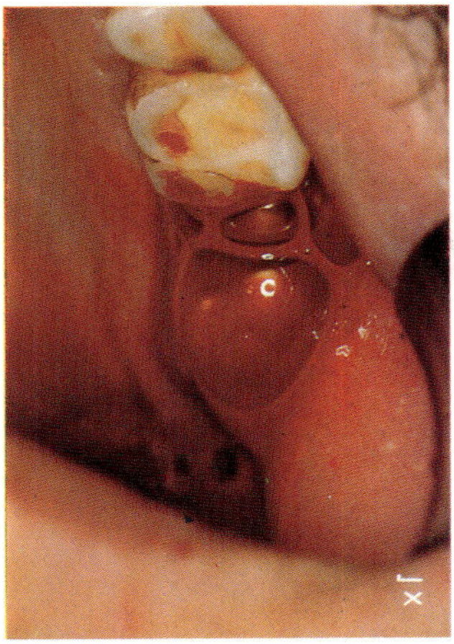

125 Positive direct nose-blowing test following surgical extraction of upper right wisdom tooth.

obviously essential to cover the defect by means of a large flap. The great loss of bone can lead to considerable difficulties in later prosthetic treatment and this might indicate a pre-prosthetic procedure such as the surgical reconstruction of the tuberosity.

Joint dislocation

A further complication during wisdom tooth extraction is unilateral or bilateral dislocation of the temporomandibular joint. The patient finds himself unable to close his mouth. On palpation and radiographic inspection, an empty fossa is found (**124**); unilateral dislocation results in displacement of the mandible towards the unaffected side.

Repositioning is achieved using the Hippocrates procedure. The operator's thumbs are protected with Mullagen and placed on the lower teeth. The other fingers grip the edge of the mandible on both sides. The mandible is then pulled forwards to allow the condyle, which is anterior to the articular eminence, to be moved below and posterior to it. In bilateral dislocation repositioning of the joints must be carried out consecutively as described above.

No further measures are necessary, since repeated dislocation is not very probable on account of post-operative care of the lower jaw and the restriction in diet. Only in the case of habitual dislocation should suitable treatment be applied after wound healing is complete (Jacobi-Hermanns and Tetsch, 1981).

6.1.5 Sinus complications

Perforation of the sinus

Perforation of the maxillary sinus during the extraction of upper wisdom teeth is a relatively frequent complication because of the close proximity of the impacted, displaced teeth to the alveolar recess of the sinus. After every tooth extraction it should be ascertained whether there is an oral-antral communication, either by a direct and indirect nose-blowing test (**125**) or in doubtful cases by careful probing of the socket. In our own practice, it occurs in 6.1% of cases. With advancing age the risk increases considerably. While up to 40 years of age a connection is diagnosed in only 3.3% of cases, the percentage in the 41–80 year age group is around 25%. If there is positive proof, tight wound closure must follow at once, as the danger of infection increases with every hour after the perforation (Lehnert and Lehmann, 1968).

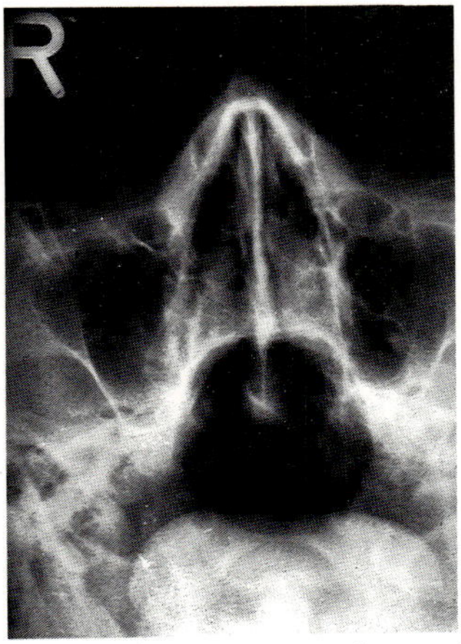

126 Nasal cavity radiograph with residual root following wisdom tooth extraction. Located in lateral sinus region.

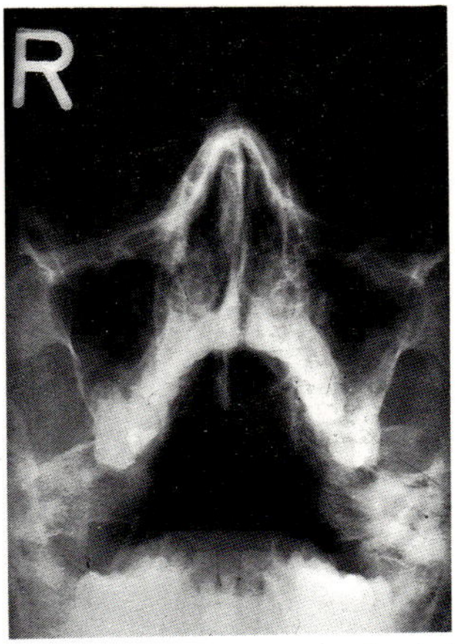

127 Residual root in the left maxillary sinus. Located in medial sinus region.

Tension-free wound closure is an important requirement for complication-free healing. Mattress or periosteal sutures following dissection of the periosteum to lengthen the vestibular mucous membrane periosteal flap (Rehrmann, 1936) can contribute to secure adaptation of the edges of the wound. These problems do not usually arise in wisdom tooth extraction as sufficient mucous membrane is available. Renewal of the edges of the wound may be necessary following extraction of partially impacted wisdom teeth.

Immediate tight covering of the defect is *omitted* only under the following exceptional circumstances:

Tooth or root in the antrum

Wisdom teeth or fractured roots are easily displaced into the maxillary sinus by rough procedures or careless use of elevators (**126, 127**). Their removal is absolutely essential because they might give rise to massive inflammatory complications, even years later. In favourable cases it is possible to undertake the removal of the tooth or root from the enlarged socket. However, alternative access, through the canine fossa, must frequently be chosen; the use of an antroscope makes this easier to locate (**128, 129;** Schmidseder and Lambrecht, 1978). The removal of tooth or root should always be left to experienced specialists. No time should be lost in these cases, in order to minimise the danger of infection.

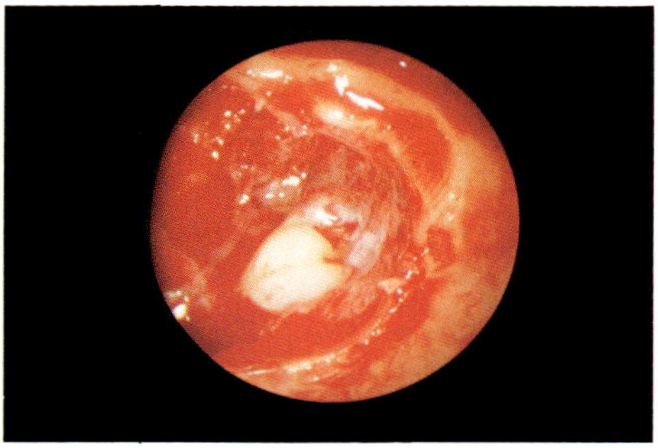

128 Endoscopic picture of a wisdom tooth luxated into the sinus.

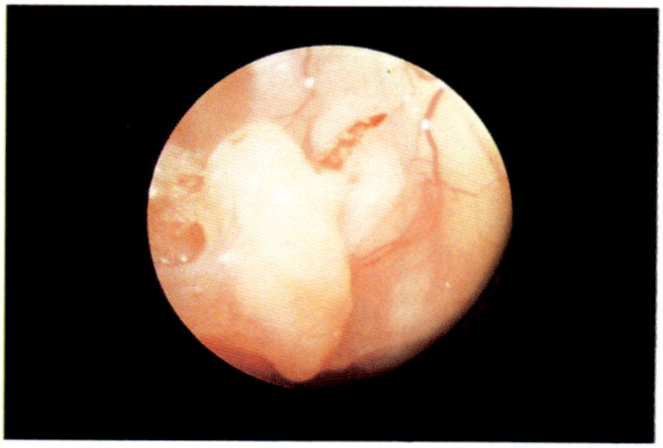

129 Endoscopic picture of a root fragment located beneath the mucous membrane of the sinus.

It is desirable, when referring the patient, to have the surgeon notified by telephone and to have the patient take the fractured tooth and radiographs along with him. Information about the type and volume of injected local anaesthetic is also important. This information prevents the maximum permissible dose of the anaesthetic being exceeded and therefore reduces the risk of a toxic reaction.

Infections of the maxillary sinus

Pus may exude from an oral–antral fistula following tooth extraction, a sure sign of empyema of the sinus. Covering of the defect must be omitted under these circumstances, as with prolapse of the buccal pad of fat, which is also a cause of chronic inflammatory changes. In these cases, the patient should be referred to a specialist who can combine the covering of the oral–antral fistula with an inspection of the sinus and if necessary with further surgical treatment.

Cysts

The diagnosis of cystic processes in the region of the upper cheek teeth is not always straightforward, since cysts develop in the sinus and are difficult to detect radiologically. Contrast media, puncture and antroscopic investigations may be necessary to diagnose them. If clear liquid flows from the sinus on tooth extraction, the diagnosis of a cyst or mucocoele is probable. In these cases also, covering is dispensed with and the patient referred for antrocystectomy, if the operation cannot be performed in the practice.

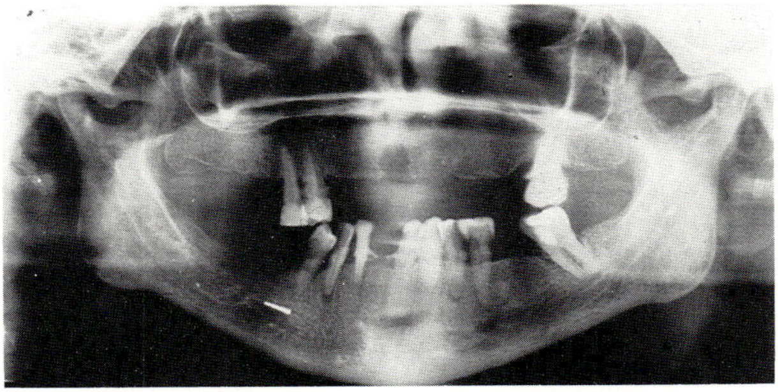

130 Radiograph with broken Lindemann bur.

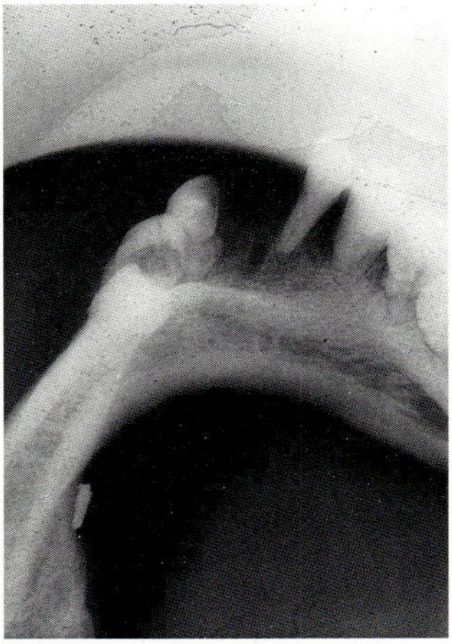

131 Lower jaw: occlusal view radiograph (see **130**).

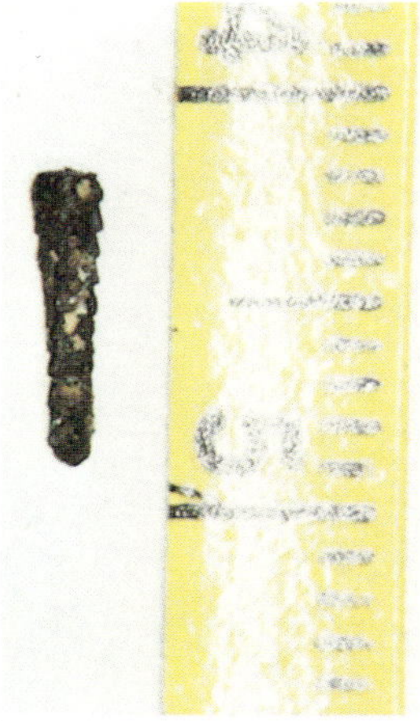

132 Extracted instrument (see **130, 131**).

Tumours

If, following extraction of a wisdom tooth with penetration of the sinus, a tumour is suspected, the patient must immediately be referred for further treatment to a specialised clinic and covering of the oral–antral communication dispensed with.

The above situations are the exception. As a rule, immediate closure of the sinus is aimed for if an oral–antral communication has been diagnosed. After the operation the patient is given, both orally and in writing, special instructions regarding after-care, which can be taken from the leaflet (see below). While antibiotic therapy is only indicated in particular cases, nose-drops to reduce swelling and, after the post-operative swelling has subsided, camomile steam inhalation should be prescribed.

If immediate closure is not carried out, inflammatory complications will certainly set in, often requiring prolonged treatment and sinus surgery.

Precautions following surgical closure of an oral-maxillary sinus communication

1. Please take note of the leaflet concerning precautions following surgical operations (see p.57-58 MS).
2. Smoking is absolutely forbidden for the following 8 days.
3. Slight nose-bleeds may occur during the next few days. You should on no account blow your nose or play a wind instrument.
4. In the following week you should take only liquid or finely minced food.
5. Apply one drop of the solution you have received into each nostril three times daily.
6. From the third day after the operation, use a camomile steam bath daily in the evening.
7. The sutures will be removed in 8–10 days.

6.1.6 Instrument breakage

Improved materials have made breakage of instruments rare but it can still happen through defective materials, frequent sterilisation and incorrect handling. Mechanical instruments must be tested thoroughly before use. Vogel (1979) describes the claims for legal liability of 12 patients in whom parts of instruments were left at the operation site; in 8 cases nearly intact bone burs and in 3 cases non-surgical burs were found in the alveolus, only 6 of these being associated with lower wisdom teeth.

Fractured burs must be removed at once because of the danger of inflammatory complications or metal poisoning. It should be kept in mind that small fragments are often very difficult to locate, as objects thought to be in the bone often turn out to be in the soft tissue. Two-dimensional radiographs help in ascertaining the precise location of the foreign body (**130–133**). The difficulty of removal is often under-estimated in these cases. The operation should therefore be left to an experienced colleague who is able to deal with any complications which may arise.

6.2 Post-operative complications

6.2.1 Infections

Infections are the most important post-operative complications, alveolitis being most common.

Alveolitis

Following a short, trouble-free period of about 2–3 days, considerable pain sets in which in the lower jaw can radiate as far as the joint and ear regions and in the upper jaw as far as the eye and temple regions. The local lymph nodes are often enlarged and tender. The patients look very ill and their general state of health is further impaired by their restricted food intake.

The causes of this post-extraction pain are numerous. The bony socket is normally protected by a blood clot which is replaced during healing, first by granulation tissue, then by connective tissue and finally by bone. If a stable clot does not form or if it breaks down through infection, an infection of the socket wall, of the so-called osteomyelitis type, occurs, together

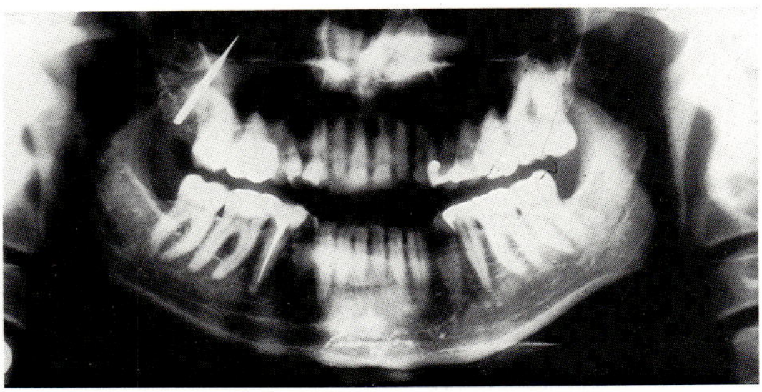

133 Broken Lindemann bur in the right maxillary sinus.

with irritation of the exposed nerve endings which gives rise to severe pain. This neuritis can spread to the inferior alveolar nerve and is then described as stem neuritis.

With the secretion of pus, separation of sequestra can occur, in extreme cases of the entire alveolar wall.

The vasoconstrictive additive in the local anaesthetic is quoted as the cause of 'dry socket'. According to Wassmund (1935) stasis occurs, followed by thrombosis, which prevents further bleeding in the reactive hyperaemic phase.

Infection of the alveolus can arise from periapical tissue following extraction in an acutely inflamed region, from infected marginal periodontium or from the oral cavity. Of these, the last seems to be the most frequent source of infection.

While alveolitis seldom occurs in the upper jaw, it is observed more frequently in the lower jaw. The following factors are responsible for this:

- retention of decay and breakdown products, food particles and saliva,
- greater surgical trauma due to the compact structure of the bone and the greater size of the teeth,
- lack of an area of fixed gingiva in the region of the wisdom tooth,
- pumping action of the masseter muscle,
- poorer blood supply to the compact bone,
- greater mechanical stress on the wound,
- lack of bony support for the wound closure,
- poor access for oral hygiene measures.

The treatment for alveolitis and post-extraction pain consists of local measures which, if applied sequentially, rapidly resolve the condition. Numerous methods of treatment have been reported; we will describe only well-established procedures here. Following removal of sutures, the bacterially decomposed blood clot is superficially removed with a sharp curette, the socket is flushed out with 3% hydrogen peroxide solution and a dressing inserted. Chlorophenol–camphor–menthol preparation (CHKM, ED84) has proved a useful medication, as in addition to its antiseptic effect, it also has local anaesthetic properties. Usually, this treatment is not very painful and can be carried out without local anaesthetic. Where there is very severe pain, anaesthesia is advisable to obtain at least temporary relief. In these extremely painful cases, the local treatment should be carried out twice daily or at even shorter intervals; the additional application of

Anaesthesin powder can accelerate the relief from pain. After the acute symptoms have subsided the application of a zinc oxide–eugenol dressing, which can be left for a longer period, is recommended.

In addition to the local treatment, an analgesic which is suited to the individual case should be prescribed. In the case of intractable pain, an I.V. injection of a potent analgesic (e.g. Fortral) may also be necessary.

Soft tissue and bone infections

Considerable trauma to the tissue, surgery in an acutely inflamed area, use of non-sterile instruments and general lack of resistance of the body often result in extensive inflammatory processes in the soft tissue. Their unfavourable location in the region of the angle of the jaw and tuberosity may lead to rapid formation of abscesses. With infection following extraction of lower wisdom teeth there is the danger of cheek, pterygomandibular, parapharyngeal, peritonsillar, sublingual, submandibular and perimandibular abscess formation.

Following extraction of a wisdom tooth from the upper jaw, abscesses are observed predominantly in the cheeks, temples, pterygopalatine fossa or the maxillary sinus. Abscesses of this sort must be lanced and drained. If there is a tendency towards spreading, antibiotic treatment is necessary.

While in our clinic no abscesses resulted from extraction of upper wisdom teeth, they occurred following osteotomy in the mandible in 1.3% of cases in the 12–14-year-olds and in 8.7% of the over-40 age group (see **81**).

Bone infections can arise haematogenically or by transfer. They rarely arise after tooth extraction but may lead to considerable therapeutic problems (**134, 135**). Especially at risk are patients who have had treatment of the jaw with ionising radiation. The primary result of irradiation is an aseptic necrosis of the bone, which usually remains clinically latent and can give rise to radio-osteomyelitis as a result of secondary infection. Teeth should therefore only be extracted if absolutely necessary and under antibiotic coverage. Sockets should be closed following the extraction - epiperiosteal covering has proved useful for this. When taking the case history, the patient must be asked about all radiotherapy to the head and neck region, since it is possible that the jaw may lie in the radiation field in cases of malignant tumours of the neck. In doubtful cases, one should refer back to the radiologist. It is better in these cases to carry out the surgical

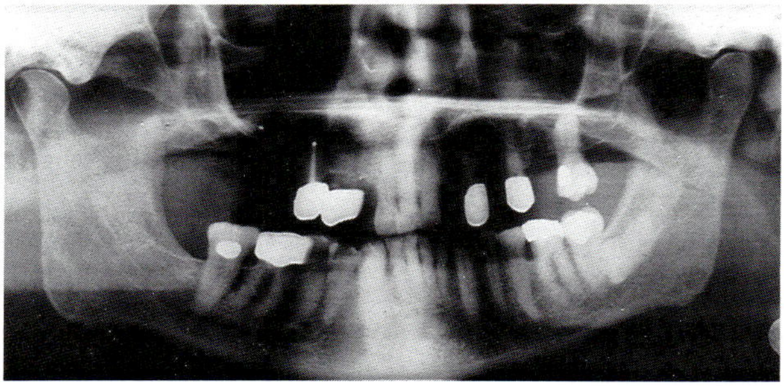

134 Horizontally displaced lower left wisdom tooth.

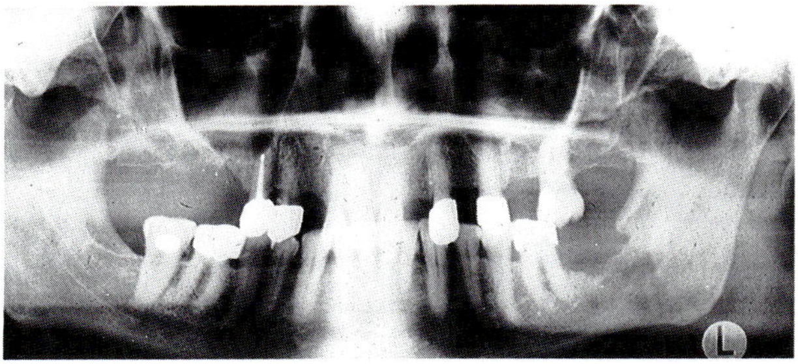

135 Osteomyelitis in the left angle following extraction of lower left second and third molars (see **134**).

removal of the teeth *before* radiotherapy.

Wound healing problems, which persist despite intensive local and general treatment, may be due to systemic disorders which had not previously been diagnosed. Especially important are haematological and metabolic disorders. A medical specialist should be consulted in these cases. Local healing problems often indicate a malignant tumour; if there is the slightest suspicion the patient should be referred to a specialist.

6.2.2 Haemorrhages

Haemorrhages following surgical extraction of wisdom teeth are manifested either as early or late bleeding. Bleeding immediately after or within a few hours of the operation is generally the result of a relative hyperaemia arising from the vasoconstriction which is in turn caused by the anaesthetic with its vasoconstrictive additive and by the surgical trauma. It can nearly always be arrested by local measures.

First, a bite swab is applied, followed by an inspection after 20 minutes. If the bleeding has not stopped by this time the wound is examined and closed tightly with mattress sutures. If this does not stop the bleeding the socket is dressed. Resorbable packs have proved effective, especially denatured cellulose (Tabotamp). As a further measure, the local application of thrombin or fibrin preparations and the placement of dressing plates is recommended. Biting on silicone impression material can also be used as a pressure dressing.

In the majority of cases the loss of blood is exaggerated by the patient. Because of the increased post-operative secretion of saliva, the loss of blood resulting from relatively slight bleeding is over-estimated. Therefore, any possible circulatory complication should be diagnosed early by taking the pulse rate and measuring blood pressure. A rapid pulse and lowering of the systolic blood pressure should be regarded as dangerous signs. In these cases I.V. infusion of a plasma expander or an electrolyte solution are indicated. The patient should not be allowed to leave the clinic until the circulatory condition has been stabilised. In the case of significant circulatory reaction the haemoglobin level should be measured.

Delayed bleeding commences 8–10 days after the operation and is the result of breakdown of clots in the blood vessels due to infection or increased fibrinolysis. Closure of the wound is contra-indicated in these cases, as wound infection is also present; open treatment with suitable dressing must be carried out.

Patients with *haemorrhagic disorders* should not be treated surgically in private practice, since fatal haemorrhages may occur. If the patient was not previously known to have a disorder of this type, and if severe bleeding occurs, one should attempt to control it with thrombin preparations and dressings and transfer him at once to a specialised hospital for diagnosis and treatment.

Anticoagulant therapy is particularly important, as the number of patients receiving this treatment is relatively large. This is a long-term therapy with coumarin derivatives and phenylindandiones, which displace vitamin K1 from the enzyme complex and thus cause diminished production of plasma clotting factors. The degree to which the blood clotting is retarded is estimated by the Quick method of partial thromboplastin time determination (PTT), in which a value of 100% represents normal clotting. The optimum therapeutic effect lies between values of 15 and 20%, since above 30% the treatment is ineffective and below 15% there is the danger of spontaneous haemorrhage. Anticoagulant therapy is used in cases of venous and arterial thrombo-embolism. Myocardial infarctions, heart valve and blood vessel replacements are the most important indications.

If surgical intervention is necessary the dentist should always consult the physician or consultant in charge of the patient and on no account alter the anticoagulant therapy himself. Every interruption of the therapy and intravenous administration of vitamin K1 is a risk since a transiently elevated clotting gradient can occur as a 'rebound effect'; the danger of an embolism or an infarction is correspondingly raised. While individual periodontally involved teeth may be extracted with the appropriate local measures – including the use of fibrin agglutinators – without altering the therapeutic PTT value, a value of 30% is necessary for surgical wisdom tooth extraction. In these cases, the risk of stopping the anticoagulant must be set against the risks which may arise from leaving the wisdom tooth in place.

Many drugs cause fairly considerable changes in tolerance towards coumarin and phenylindandione. A lowering of the coumarin tolerance – and hence a corresponding danger of haemorrhage – is brought about by salicylic acid derivatives,

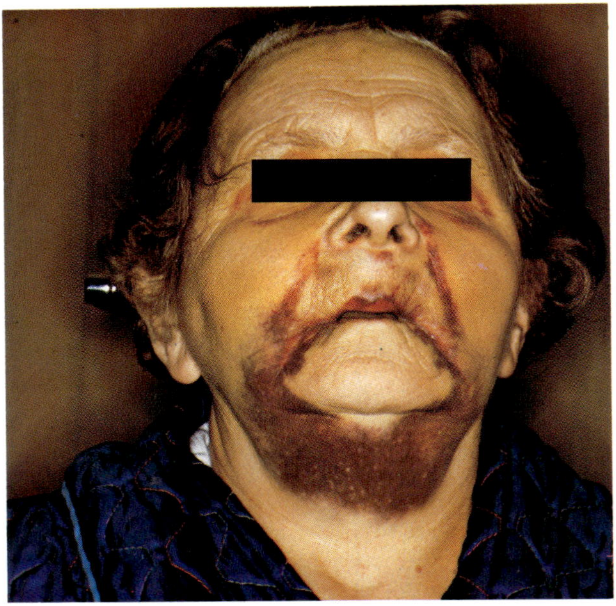

136 Extensive haematoma following wisdom tooth extraction in a case of thrombocytopathy.

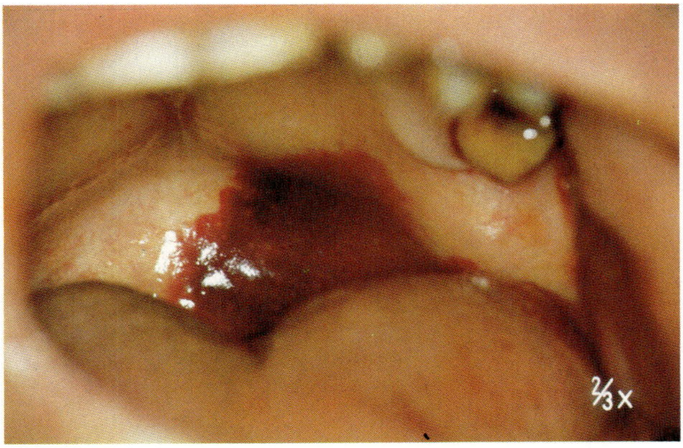

137 Haematoma of the soft palate following palatal injection.

phenylbutazone and all the broad-spectrum antibiotics acting against *E. coli* which destroy the vitamin K1-producing intestinal commensals. Therefore it is of prime importance to ensure that all mixed analgesics containing salicylic acid derivatives are avoided.

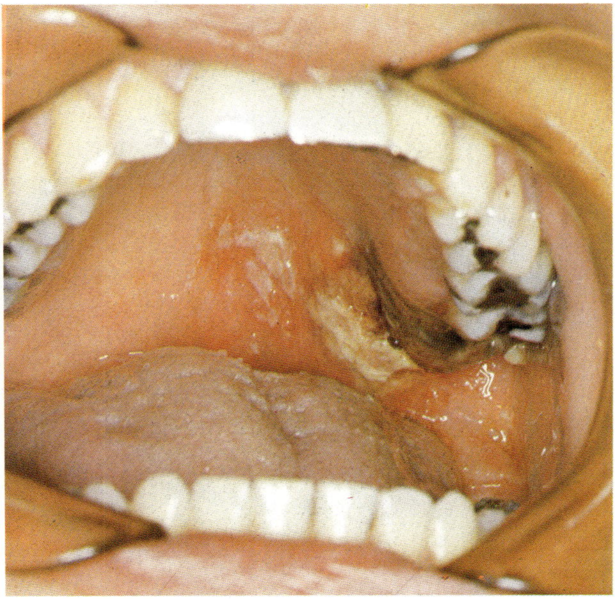

138 Extensive necrosis of the mucous membrane following palatal injection for extraction of the upper left third molar.

An increase in coumarin tolerance, which is associated with a danger of thrombosis, can be produced by preparations containing vitamin K1, atropine, adrenalin, barbiturates and some psycho-pharmaceuticals. It is advisable to have PTT values determined before, during and after surgery.

6.2.3 Haematomas

Post-operative haematomas are common and should be treated according to their extent and location; often the use of cold compresses is sufficient. Resorption may be accelerated by the early application of varidase or heparin-containing ointments. There is increased danger of infection, which may justify antibiotic therapy.

Where bruising is very extensive, the possibility of a thrombocytopathy or vasopathy must be considered (**136, 137**). In every case a clotting analysis should be carried out.

6.2.4 Necrosis of the mucous membrane

Poor injection technique, incorrect surgical procedure and neglect of after-care by the patient can lead to necrosis of the mucosa, which retards wound healing and leads to considerable problems.

Palatal injection with a maximum of 0.2 ml of anaesthetic solution should be carried out without the use of excess pressure lest the blood supply be damaged and pressure necroses arise (**138**). This holds also for incisions in which the flap base is made too narrow or for damage to soft tissue caused by faulty technique. Damage through biting or hot food burns before the anaesthetic has worn off also frequently results in necrosis of the mucosa. Treatment of such conditions consists of local measures. Careful cleaning with hydrogen peroxide solution, rinsing with camomile and, if necessary, application of adhesive cortisone-containing ointments is advised.

If necrosis occurs spontaneously one should always suspect a systemic disorder (e.g. diabetes mellitus, leukaemia, agranulocytosis).

7 SURGICAL EXTRACTION OF WISDOM TEETH IN HIGH-RISK PATIENTS

More complications are expected with high-risk patients. Certain disorders (infectious diseases) can result in danger to the patient himself or to other people. They always require special care and necessitate the taking of precautions or transfer to a hospital.

The most important measure for the *prevention of emergencies* is to acquire knowledge of the risk factors by careful taking of the case history and in doubtful cases by consulting the physician in charge. Other preventive measures include psychological preparation and guidance of the patient, reasonable premedication, choice of suitable anaesthetic, calculation of the maximum permissible dose for the individual and correct injection technique.

Since emergencies cannot be excluded in spite of all precautions taken, preparatory measures for such events should be instituted in every practice. These include the preparation of emergency apparatus and drugs (preferably in an emergency box) and emergency numbers (doctor, hospital, ambulance, taxi) next to the telephone. For mastery of unforeseen incidents, constant revision of the basic groundwork and training for emergencies (re-motivation) are certainly the most important requirements. Such courses are run by numerous organisations and are regularly announced in the further education programmes of dental associations.

The most important problem groups from the point of view of dental surgical operations are given below.

7.1 Cardiovascular diseases

In this group are included a large number of different diseases (Table 9). In acute disease states, the indication for wisdom tooth extraction must be very carefully established in every case. One should avoid the addition of a vasoconstrictor to the local anaesthetic, since in conjunction with the endogenously released catecholamines it may cause circulatory complications. Hypotonic patients are an exception, as an increase in vascular

Table 9 Local anaesthesia (LA) for cardiovascular disorders

Problem group	LA type	Vaso-constrictor	Sedation	Other
Cardiac insufficiency	Amide	Without	Tranquilliser (e.g. Valium 5-10 mg)	
Coronary artery insufficiency	Amide	Without	Tranquilliser	
Arrhythmias	Amide	Without	Tranquilliser	beta-blocker for tachycardia
Myocardial infarction	Amide	Without	Tranquilliser	
Stroke	Amide	Without	Tranquilliser	
Hypotension	Amide	With		Sympathetico-mimetic (e.g. Effortil)
Hypertension	Amide	Without		Possibly beta-blockers (e.g. Aptin, Visken)

tone, with corresponding rise in blood pressure, is desirable in their case.

General sedation of the patient by means of premedication leads to a reduction in endogenous adrenalin release and can be regarded as a sensible measure for the prevention of complications. With sufficient experience and with attention to the contra-indications (e.g. bronchial asthma, bradycardia, cardiac insufficiency, hypotension, diabetes mellitus) the pre-surgical prescription of a beta-blocker may be advisable (e.g. Aptin 25 mg, Visken 5 mg) where there is tachycardia and hypertension.

With high-risk patients in this category, it is advisable to conduct the operation under ECG surveillance and with an I.V. drip, in order to detect complications in good time and to be able to treat them. These measures must be carried out in a hospital so that supervision by appropriate specialists (anaesthetists, for example) is possible.

The particular problems associated with coumarin therapy following myocardial infarction, cardiac surgery, embolisms or strokes have already been discussed in Section 6.2.2.

Patients with an implanted pacemaker do not run any particular risk these days, since trouble-free Demand-pacemakers are inserted almost exclusively. In doubtful cases, any disruption (e.g. by electrotome) is avoided by covering with a lead shield.

7.2 Endocrine disorders

In this category, diabetes mellitus and hyperthyroidism are of most interest.

Diabetes mellitus

About 3% of the population are diabetic. This insulin deficiency can be divided into two types:

Type I – Juvenile, insulin-requiring diabetes mellitus.

Type II – Maturity onset diabetes, not requiring insulin.

Infections of the gingivae, ulceration of the oral mucosa, angular cheilosis, progressive periodontal disease and dryness of the mouth are diagnostic features of diabetes mellitus (**139**).

The risks of a surgical operation lie in the possibility of loss of metabolic control resulting in hyper- or hyopoglycaemic crisis, in increased tendency towards haemorrhage and occurrence of wound healing problems.

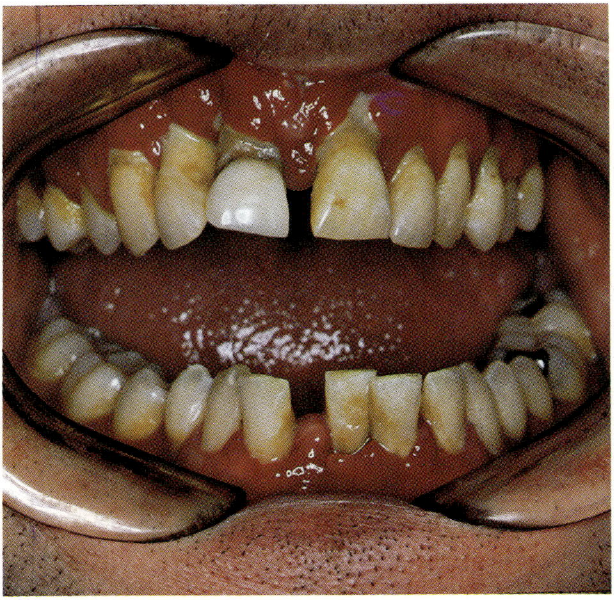

139 Progressively developing periodontitis in a juvenile insulin-dependent diabetic (Type I).

Potential causes of loss of metabolic control are stress situations, local anaesthesia if a preparation containing adrenalin is injected, post-operative medication, pre- and post-operative changes in diet and changes in drug therapy. If a wisdom tooth extraction is planned, it should be emphasised to the patient, when he is told the date of the operation, that he should not alter his medication and diet and above all should not arrive on the day on an empty stomach. In our experience there is a widespread belief that fasting is necessary even for operations under local anaesthesia. For a diabetic who has injected himself with insulin the lack of food will certainly lead to a hypoglycaemic crisis.

Juvenile insulin-dependent diabetics are particularly prone to going out of control, besides which they frequently show great fluctuations in blood sugar level. Special care is needed here and cooperation with the physician, consultant or hospital is absolutely essential. This also holds for the pre-operative preparation and the post-operative care of the patient. Following an intra-oral operation a change in diet is usually necessary and this can have a considerable effect on blood sugar level. The general practitioner or consultant should be consulted about the advisability of admitting the patient to hospital.

Increased tendency to haemorrhage can be attributed to vasopathy and frequently recurring infection of the oral mucosa. Bleeding during or after the operation can usually be controlled by local measures.

Increased incidence of infection is caused by impairment of antibody production arising from lack of glycogen; vasopathy is another factor. Infections harmless in themselves can affect the insulin requirements. In addition to conservative surgical procedure and wound drainage, prophylactic antibiotic therapy should be considered.

Surgical operations should be carried out in the morning after breakfast, since at this time the metabolic state is relatively stable. The beginning of the week is preferable to the end in order to ensure post-operative surveillance by a suitable specialist.

With reference to local anaesthesia, it should be observed that injected adrenalin is antagonistic to insulin and therefore should not be used in diabetics. A local anaesthetic without vasoconstrictive additive is advised.

The problem of post-operative analgesia has already been considered in Section 4.6.4.

If, in spite of all precautions, the metabolism does go out of

Table 10 Operative procedure in diabetics

Thorough case history
Consultation with physician or hospital doctor (assurance of peri-operative control of blood sugar level)
Hospitalisation in case of severely fluctuating blood sugar levels
Operation at the beginning of the week
Operation after breakfast
No change in medication by patient or surgeon
No alteration in diet
Local anaesthetic without vasoconstrictive additive
Conservative operative technique
No salicylates or pyrazolone derivatives
Post-operative blood sugar control by the physician in charge
Possibly antibiotic coverage

control, differentiation between hypo- and hyperglycaemic crisis is not easy for the inexperienced. As a rule, the patient himself recognises the onset of hypoglycaemia; it is easily and effectively treated by taking sugar orally. However, with considerable fluctuations of blood sugar level, sudden loss of consciousness may occur, in which case an intravenous injection (40–80 ml) of a 40% glucose solution is necessary. This treatment is correct for hypoglycaemic shock and will not have any noticeable adverse effect in the case of hyperglycaemic coma.

Hyperthyroidism

In the case of overactivity of the thyroid gland, the addition of adrenalin to the local anaesthetic should be avoided, since in conjunction with the endogenous release of adrenalin, a thyrotoxic crisis may occur. The symptoms consist of marked restlessness, stupor, a feeling of disorientation, raised temperature (more than 40°C), increased pulse rate (more than 140/min., arrhythmias) and disturbance of cerebral function. Treatment consists of sedation, giving oxygen, cortisone injections and finally admission to hospital.

7.3 Liver diseases

The amide-type local anaesthetics predominantly in use today (e.g. lidocaine, mepivacaine, carticain) are broken down in the liver by microsomal enzymes which split the amide bond. This breakdown takes place relatively slowly and leads to higher blood levels than with local anaesthetics of the ester type. This increases the danger of accumulation if subsequent injections are administered. The maximum permissible dose should therefore be regarded as the maximum dose for the day. In the case of chronic liver disease (e.g. cirrhosis of the liver) a preparation of the ester type (e.g. Novocain) should be used, since the liver burden is considerably reduced as a result of significant breakdown in the tissues and blood, and the danger of accumulation is reduced.

With restricted liver function an increased tendency to haemorrhage is to be expected, which should be investigated before surgery.

7.4 Kidney diseases

Among these diseases, those which are connected with restricted renal function and which may result in chronic renal failure are of importance in oral surgery. Treatment with drugs will be considered first. All substances which are excreted via the kidneys must be used only after consultation with the specialist, as the danger of accumulation is particularly high. Hypertonia should be suspected with kidney disease.

Renal failure necessitates dialysis to remove urinary substances (creatine, creatinine, urea, uric acid) and fluid, and to maintain electrolyte balance. Generally, extracorporeal haemodialysis is used (also as home dialysis), in which every two or three days the heparinised blood is passed for several hours through a filter system which removes urinary substances and fluid. The heparinisation forbids surgical operation within a period of 6 hours after dialysis has finished. The best time is on the day following dialysis. Since dialysis, and occasionally heparinisation, must usually be repeated on the first or second day after surgery, wound closure should be very tight to reduce the risk of a post-operative haemorrhage.

In addition to the danger of hepatitis (see Section 7.8), *renal osteopathy* must also be suspected in long-term dialysis patients. Osteolytic processes may occur in the jaw region as a result of disturbance of calcium and phosphate metabolism (Machtens *et al.*, 1974) and may result in dissolution of the lamina dura of the sockets and the root apices of caries-free teeth. This is often erroneously diagnosed as apical osteitis and wrongly treated as such. On the other hand, sclerosis can considerably complicate surgical procedure. If the bone has been previously damaged in this way, a greater risk of infection is to be expected.

7.5 Bronchial asthma

Asthma attacks may be induced by psychological causes and frequently occur during dental treatment. The use of a local anaesthetic with a high level of adrenalin is expected, since this stimulates the beta-receptors and produces broncho-dilation. Beta-blockers are contra-indicated for asthmatics but a psycho-sedative may be advisable. The attack itself is treated with aerosol sprays (e.g. Berotec).

7.6 Epilepsy

Epileptic seizures may be induced by exogenous or endogenous adrenalin influx. These patients should be treated with local anaesthetics without vasoconstrictive additives. Regardless of the type of operation, one should make sure that the drug therapy for the basic ailment is not interrupted, or is only changed by the neurologist in charge of the case.

7.7 Pregnancy

Surgical extraction of wisdom teeth during pregnancy is only necessary in rare cases. As a rule, it is possible to postpone the operation by use of local measures. If this treatment does not alleviate the problems, the operation should be undertaken, if possible, during the second trimester of pregnancy as there is less risk during this period. No posterior pituitary hormones (Octapressin) should be used as vasoconstrictors as these may cause contraction of the uterus and induce the onset of labour. Xylonest or Anaesthesin should not be used on account of the danger of methaemoglobin formation. A local anaesthetic of the

Table 11 Local anaesthesia (LA) in problem patients

Problem group	LA type	Vasoconstrictor	Sedation
Diabetes mellitus	Amide	Without	—
Hyperthyroidism	Amide	Without	Tranquilliser (e.g. Valium 5–10 mg)
Liver disease	Ester	With	—
Bronchial asthma	Amide	With (high level)	Tranquilliser
Epilepsy	Amide	Without	By neurologist
Pregnancy	Amide (no Xylonest or Anaesthesin)	With	—

amide type with vasoconstrictive supplement is suitable. Additional medication should be used cautiously and critically (Fesseler, 1982).

7.8 Infectious diseases

The most important diseases in this group are hepatitis and tuberculosis; they can endanger staff and subsequent patients. If one of these infectious diseases is known to be present, suitable precautions should be observed. Unfortunately, there are a large number of undiagnosed cases and this represents the real problem. Treatment of infectious patients should be left to the end of the day and contact with other patients prevented as far as possible. In addition, special disinfection measures are essential which prelude the immediate treatment of another patient in the same room.

Hepatitis

The incidence of hepatitis is 5–6 times higher in dentists than in the general population. In the surgical profession, it is even worse. The incidence of the disease increases considerably with age. Hepatitis is a disease that has to be reported to the health authorities and is recognised as an occupational disease of dentists without further proof. However, if a patient with one of these diseases is treated, the fact should always be recorded. This is especially true of those cases in which there has been injury to the surgeon.

Inflammation of the liver is brought about by a series of different viruses with hepatotropic properties. Hepatitis A virus and Hepatitis B virus are hepatitis viruses in the strict sense. In addition, Non A/Non B hepatitis viruses have been described. About 25 000 cases are recorded annually in Germany. However, since only an estimated 10–25% of all cases are reported, and many cases remain clinically undiagnosed, a much higher morbidity must be assumed. Hepatitis B plays a crucial role in dental practice.

Hepatitis B virus, i.e. HBsAg (Hepatitis B-surface-antigen), is principally transmitted by blood or blood derivatives but is also found in secretions and excreted substances (e.g. in saliva and tears). Although these have a lower concentration of antigen compared with blood, infection from them is possible. The incubation time is highly variable, ranging from 60 to 160 days. In many cases, hepatitis develops without icterus and without clinical signs. Frequently the only symptoms are weakness and fatigue.

Active immunisation is being developed at present and will be available in the near future (Hevac B Pasteur, H-B-Vax). Specific treatment previously has consisted of passive immunisation with anti-HBs antibodies. Specific anti-HBs immunoglobulins with high antibody titre are able to prevent hepatitis B with a high degree of certainty. In the case of contact with a wound, the immunoglobulin should be injected intramuscularly within 12 hours, at a dose rate of 0.04–0.06 ml/kg body weight. Protection by this passive immunisation lasts for 2–5 months. The injections must be repeated after 4–6 weeks and 8–12 weeks. Prophylactic measures to be observed with sick patients or hepatitis-risk patients are particularly important (Table 12).

Table 12 Hepatitis-risk patients

Physicians, dentists
Medical technicians
Hospital and surgery staff
Dialysis patients
Patients receiving long-term hospital treatment
Drug addicts
Prostitutes
Homosexuals
Alcoholics
Tramps and vagrants

Personal hygiene must be the principal measure for the doctor or dentist in charge of the case and for his assistants. Frequent hand washing and the use of disposable gloves can prevent further spread of the virus. A preparation is available which within a short time period (2 minutes) brings about a complete alteration and disintegration of the hepatitis B virus; this is the hand disinfecting agent Primasept M. Virus disinfection is also of prime importance; physical and chemical methods are suitable for virus inactivation. The most effective methods are burning of infectious material, dry heat sterilisation (160°C for 120 minutes) and steam autoclaving (120°C at 1.1 atmospheres for 15 minutes).

For disinfection of contaminated areas of skin or delicate apparatus, which cannot be sterilised, chemical disinfectants, for which there must be proof of hepatitis B virocidal activity (e.g. Gigasept, formaldehyde, Lysoformin), come under consideration.

Objects in the operating room which are not in use should be covered. The surgical team must wear protective clothing, as described in Section 4.3 (**140**). Contaminated instruments should generally be disinfected *before* cleaning.

Tuberculosis

Tuberculosis is an infectious granulomatous inflammatory condition which is caused by a mycobacterium. Like hepatitis it has to be reported to the health authorities. An extensive study by Seeliger and Gebhardt (1978), based on 5433 autopsies, revealed that 3.7% of cases had severe tuberculosis, of which only 51.3% had been unequivocally diagnosed clinically. It is supposed that 5% of patients over 60 years of age have an undiagnosed open tuberculosis of the lungs. On the basis of official statistics concerning tuberculosis, it used to be thought that the reduced risk to children these days made BCG immunisation superfluous. BCG protective vaccination was recommended only as an individual protective measure in special isolated cases, if there was a risk to neonates from their environment. From 1975 to 1977 the vaccine was not generally available. In the course of these two years, when no vaccination was performed, the incidence amongst children increased abruptly. About 1000 children in West Germany became ill – about ten times as many as had been predicted. Therefore, paediatricians nowadays advocate renewed official recommendation of BCG vaccination.

In known cases of tuberculosis and high-risk patients, the same

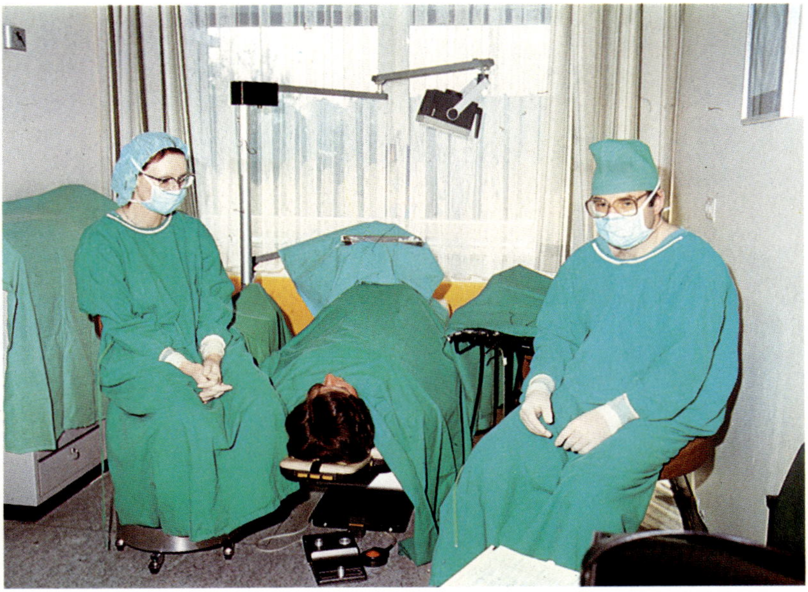

140 Dental treatment of a hepatitis patient. Treatment chair, patient and all items not required are covered. Use of a tray for all instruments required. Protective clothing: gown, cap and mask, gloves, protective glasses.

hygienic measures should be observed as have been described for hepatitis.

These comments should make it clear that the real danger, to surgeon, staff and subsequent patients, of infectious diseases lies in the unknown number of undiagnosed cases.

Literature

Literature

Aderhold, L. and G. Frenkel: Die Aufklärung in der zahnärztlichen Chirurgie. *Zahnärztl. Praxis* 32, 184 (1981)

App, G. R. and R. J. Stephens: Parodontale Aspekte impaktierter Zähne. In: Slaughter, T. W. and L. J. Boucher, Impaktierte Zähne, okklusale Artikulation. Medica, Stuttgart (1980)

Becker, R.: Beobachtung über die Zunahme der Kieferosteomyelitis und Änderung ihres Krankheitsbildes. *Dtsch. zahnärztl. Z.* 14, 1373 (1959)

Becker, R.: Zur Klinik und Therapie des unteren Weisheitszahnes. *Dtsch. Zahnärztekalender* (1961)

Becker, R.: Zysten im Kiefer- und Gesichtsbereich. In: Haunfelder, D., L. Hupfauf, W. Ketterl and G. Schmuth, *Praxis der Zahnheilkunde.* Urban & Schwarzenberg, Munich (1970)

Becker, R. and R. Katterbach: Bewährte Instrumente und Hilfsmittel in der zahnärztlichen Chirurgie. *Dtsch. Zahnärztebl.* 21, 91 (1967)

Bethmann, W. and O. Krüger: Zur Dentitio difficilis. *Dtsch. Stomatol.* 16, 401 (1966)

Bohmer, H.: Verlagerte Weisheitszähne im aufsteigenden Ast des Unterkiefers. *Zahnärztl. Welt* 56, 65 (1955)

Calais, P.: Retinierte Zähne im Alterskiefer und Probleme bei ihrer Entfernung. *Dtsch. zahnärztl. Z.* 2, 171 (1970)

Celesnik, F.: Indikationen für die Entfernung retinierter Zähne. *Öst. Z. Stomat.* 1, 7 (1971)

Dachi, S. F. and F. V. Howell: A survey of 3874 routine full-mouth radiographs. III. A study of impacted teeth. *Oral Surg.* 14, 1165 (1961)

Donovan, M. H.: Occlusal radiography of the mandibular third molar. *Dent. Radiogr. Photogr.* 25, 53 (1952)

Engelhardt, J. P. and L. Grün: Hygienemassnahmen in der Zahnärztpraxis. *Zahnärztl. Mitt.* 71, 1258 (1981)

Eschler, J.: Die operative Entfernung retinierter Zähne. *Zahnärztl. Prax.* 18, 145 (1967)

Eskici, A.: Replantation und Transplantation von Zähnen und Zahnkeimen. *Dtsch. zahnärztl. Z.* 35, 343 (1980)

Freitag, V.: Komplikationshäufigkeit nach Weisheitszahnentfernung. *Dtsch. zahnärztl. Z.* 22, 1030 (1967)

Frenkel, G.: Das Gutachten bei Verletzungen des Nervus lingualis. *Dtsch. zahnärztl. Z.* 35, 199 (1980)

Fry, K. W.: The third molar. *Brit. dent. J.* 54, 384 (1933)

Gabka, J. and H. Harnisch: *Komplikationen und Fehler bei der zahnärztlichen Behandlung.* Thieme, Stuttgart (1974)

Geheb, H.: Studie über Approximalabrasion. *Quintessenz* 32, Ref. Nr. 6248, 1405 (1981)

Günther, H.: Forensische Fragen in der Zahnheilkunde. In: Haunfelder, D., L. Hupfauf, W. Ketterl and G. Schmuth, *Praxis der Zahnheilkunde.* Urban & Schwarzenberg, Munich (1969)

Hall, R. M.: Surgical removal of impacted teeth using air turbine unit. *J. Oral. Surg., Anesth. Hosp. D. Serv.* 17, 3 (1959)

Hammer, H.: Beiträge zur Frage des Durchbruches der unteren Weisheitszähne. *Dtsch. Mschr. Zahnheilk.* 48, 265 (1930)

Harnisch, H.: *Die Durchbruchsstörungen der Weisheitszähne.* Fischer, Jena (1947)

Haunfelder, D.: Retinierte Zähne und angrenzende Tumoren (Zugleich ein Beitrag zur Frage der Entfernung retinierter Zähne). *Dtsch. zahnärztl. Z.* 19, 865 (1964)

Haunfelder, D.: Klinik und Therapie des retinierten Zahnes. In: Haunfelder, D., L. Hupfauf, W. Ketterl and G. Schmuth, *Praxis der Zahnheilkunde.* Urban & Schwarzenberg, Munich (1968)

Haunfelder, D. and P. Tetsch: Unterkieferfrakturen im Rahmen von Zahnextraktionen. *Dtsch. zahnärztl. Z.* 27, 881 (1972)

Haunfelder D. and H. Reich: Stomatologisch bedeutsame Syndrome. In: Haunfelder, D., L. Hupfauf, W. Ketterl and G. Schmuth, *Praxis der Zahnheilkunde.* Urban & Schwarzenberg, Munich (1980)

Herz, P.: *Komplikationen bei der Weisheitszahnentfernung.* Med. Diss. Mainz (1982)

Hofer, O., E. Reichenbach, Th. Spreter von Kreudenstein and E. Wannenmacher: *Lehrbuch der klinischen Zahn-, Mund- und Kieferheilkunde* Vol. 1. Barth, Leipzig (1968)

Hoppe, W.: Die odontogenen Eiterungen. In: Haunfelder, D., L. Hupfauf, W. Ketterl and G. Schmuth, *Praxis der Zahnheilkunde.* Urban & Schwarzenberg, Munich (1971)

Hunt, P. R.: Sicherheitsgesichtspunkte bei der lingualen Unterkieferchirurgie. *Quintessenz* 32, Ref. Nr. 6191, 307 (1981)

Jacobi-Hermanns, E. and P. Tetsch: Die perikapsuläre Eigenblutinjektion als Therapie der habituellen Kiefergelenkluxation. *Dtsch. zahnärztl. Z.* 36, 187 (1981)

James, W. W.: An improved procedure for the removal of impacted mandibular third molars. *Proc. R. Soc. Med.* Lond. 29, 85 (1935)

Kaminishi, R. M., W. H. Davis and N. E. Nelson: Die chirurgische Entfernung impaktierter dritter Unterkiefermolaren. In: Slaughter, T. W. and L. J. Boucher, *Impaktierte Zähne, okklusale Artikulation.* Medica, Stuttgart (1980)

Killey, H., D. C. and L. W. Kay: *The impacted wisdom tooth.* Livingstone, London (1965)

Kilpatrick, H. C. and N. Y. Yonkers: Removal of impacted third molars utilizing speeds up to 200 000 R.P.M. *Oral Surg.* 11, 364 (1958)

Kirschner, H.: Experimente mit Aluminiumoxid-Keramik. *Dtsch. zahnärztl. Z.* 36, 274 (1981)

Kirschner, H., U. Bolz, S. Enomoto, R. W. Huttemann, W. Meinel and J. Sturm: Eine neue Methode kombinierter allo-autoplastischer Zahnreplantation mit partieller Al_2O_3-Keramikwurzel. *Dtsch. zahnärztl. Z.* 33, 594 (1978)

Kirschner, H., W. Meyer, V. Bolz and K. Kalweit: Innengekühlte Bohrer und Fräsen für die Knochenchirurgie in der Zahn-, Mund- und Kieferheilkunde. *Electromedica* 3, 110 (1976)

Kirschner, H. and W. Meyer: Entwicklung einer Innenkühlung für chirurgische Bohrer. *Dtsch. zahnärztl. Z.* 30, 436 (1975)

Krekeler, G., F. Scharf and D. Tröndle: Röntgenstatistische Untersuchungen über Nichtanlage und Dystopien der Weisheitszähne. *Dtsch. zahnärztl. Z.* 29, 591 (1974)

Krüger, E.: *Operationslehre für Zahnärzte.* Quintessenz, Berlin (1976)

Kuhr, H. W. and B. Wetzstein: Entwicklung und Durchbruch der Weisheitszähne bei Fehlen von Seitenzähnen. *Fortschr. Kieferorthop.* 31, 57 (1970)

Lehnert, S. and J. Lehmann: Die Eröffnung der Kieferhöhle nach Zahnextraktion. Statistische Auswertung von 215 Fällen. *Dtsch. Zahnärztebl.* 22, 7 (1968)

Lentrodt, J. and H. G. Bull: Tierexperimentelle Untersuchungen zur Frage der Gewebsschädigung durch höchsttouriges Bohren und Fräsen im Knochen. *Dtsch. zahnärztl. Z.* 29, 230 (1974)

Lentrodt, J. and H. G. Bull: Tierexperimentelle Untersuchungen zur Frage der Knochenregeneration nach Bohrvorgängen im Knochen. *Dtsch. zahnärztl. Z.* 31, 115 (1976)

Lytle, J. J.: Indikationen und Kontraindikationen der Entfernung impaktierter Zähne. In: Slaughter, T. W. and L. J. Boucher, *Impaktierte Zähne, okklusale Artikulation.* Medica, Stuttgart (1980)

Machtens, E., E. Hjörting-Hansen, H. J. Schmallenbach and L. Werz: Keratozyste — Ameloblastom, ein klinisch diagnostisches Problem. *Dtsch. Zahn-, Mund-, Kieferheilk.* 28, 157 (1972)

Metz, H. J. and J. Lentrodt: Ausbreitung odontogener Entzündungen. *Dtsch. zahnärztl. Z.* 23, 605 (1968)

Motsch, A.: *Funktionsorientierte Einschleiftechnik für das natürliche Gebiss.* Hanser, Munich (1977)

Müller, W.: Replantation und Transplantation von Zähnen. In: Schwenzer, N. and G. Grimm, *Zahn-, Mund- und Kieferheilkunde,* Vol. 2, *Spezielle Chirurgie.* Thieme, Stuttgart (1981)

Müller, W.: Zahnentfernung. In: Schwenzer, N. and G. Grimm, *Zahn-, Mund- und Kieferheilkunde,* Vol. 2, *Spezielle Chirurgie.* Thieme, Stuttgart (1981)

Neuner, M.: *Gesichtsemphyseme in Verbindung mit zahnärztlichen Behandlungsmassnahmen und Traumen.* Med. Diss. Mainz (1977)

Pape, H.-D. and K. Ikemura: Erhebung zur prophylaktischen Entfernung der Weisheitszahnkeime. *Dtsch. zahnärztl. Z.* 34, 213 (1979)

Partsch, C.: Zur Behandlung der Kieferzysten. *Dtsch. Mschr. Zahnheilk.* 28, 252 (1910)

Plischko, M.: *Untersuchungen zur Symptomatologie und Pathologie dystopischer Zähne unter Berücksichtigung ihrer Auswirkung auf den Gesamtorganismus.* Med. Diss. Munich (1978)

Racey, G. L. and W. R. Wallace: Die chirurgische Entfernung impaktierter dritter Oberkiefermolaren. In: Slaughter, T. W. and L. J. Boucher, *Impaktierte Zähne, okklusale Artikulation.* Medica, Stuttgart (1980)

Rehrmann, A.: Eine Methode zur Schliessung von Kieferhöhlenperforationen. *Dtsch. zahnärztl. Wschr.* 39, 1136 (1936)

Ricketts, R. M.: Prognostische Untersuchungen zur Entfernung dritter Unterkiefermolaren. In: Slaughter, T. W. and L. J. Boucher, *Impaktierte Zähne, okklusale Artikulation.* Medica, Stuttgart (1980)

Ritter, W.: Röntgenuntersuchung der Zähne, der Kiefer und des Gesichtsskelettes. In: Schwenzer, N. and G. Grimm, *Zahn-, Mund- und Kieferheilkunde.* Vol. 1, Thieme, Stuttgart (1981)

Rud, J.: The split bone technique in removal of impacted mandibular third molars. *Brit. J. Oral Surg.* 28, 416 (1970)

Scheunemann, H. and J. E. Hausamen: Gutachterliche Erfahrungen bei Verletzung des Nervus lingualis mit zahnärztlich-chirurgischen Eingriffen. *Dtsch. zahnärztl. Z.* 35, 196 (1980)

Scheunemann, H. and W. Wagner: Zur Erreger- und Resistenzsituation bei Wundheilungsstörungen in der Kiefer- und Gesichtschirurgie. In: Probst, J.: *15, Jahrestagung der Deutschen Gesellschaft für plastische und Wiederherstellungschirurgie.* Springer, Berlin (1980)

Schuchardt, K., A. Eckstein and S. Lehnert: Beobachtungen und Erfahrungen bei der Diagnose und Therapie von 3591 klinisch behandelten Fällen odontogener Entzündungen im Kiefer- und Gesichtsbereich. In: Schuchardt, K., *Fortschritte der Kiefer-und Gesichtschirurgie,* Vol. IX. Thieme, Stuttgart (1964)

Schulte, W.: Die Eigenblutfüllung: Eine neue Methode zur Versorgung grösserer Knochendefekte nach intraoralen Eingriffen. *Dtsch. zahnärztl. Z.* 15, 910 (1960)

Schulz, P.: Die Verletzungen des Nervus lingualis. *Dtsch. Zahnärztekalender* (1981)

Schwarze, C. W.: The influence of third molar germectomy — a comparative long-term study. *Trans. 3rd. Int. Orthodontic Congress* (1973)

Schwarze, C. W.: Hat die Keimentfernung der Weisheitszähne Einfluss auf die Spätform des Zahnbogens? *Fortschr. Kieferorthop.* 34, 387 (1973)

Shanley, L. S.: The influence of mandibular third molars on mandibular anterior teeth. *Am. J. Orthodont.* 48, 786 (1962)

Shulman, L. B.: Impaktierte und nicht durchgetretene Zähne als Transplantat. In: Slaughter, T. W. and L. J. Boucher, *Impaktierte Zähne, okklusale Artikulation.* Medica, Stuttgart (1980)

Strukmeier, A. and H. D. Pape: Vergleichende Untersuchungen zur vestibulären und lingualen Osteotomie bei der Entfernung unterer Weisheitszähne. *Dtsch. zahnärztl. Z.* 35, 124 (1980)

Tetsch, P., H. J. Schmallenbach and E. Sabinski: Die posttraumatische Unterkieferosteomyelitis. *Dtsch. zahnärztl. Z.* 27, 895 (1972)

Tetsch, P. and W. Schneider: Innengekühlte Bohrer und Fräsen in der zahnärztlichen Chirurgie. *Dtsch. Z. Mund-Kiefer-Gesichtschir.* 1, 118 (1977)

Tetsch, P. and W. Wagner: Die Messungen des Blutdruckes in der zahnärztlichen Praxis. *Zahnärztl. Mitt.* 69, 746 (1979)

Trauner, R.: Die Entfernung retinierter Zähne. In: Pichler, H. and R. Trauner, *Kieferund Gesichtschirurgie,* Vol. I, Urban & Schwarzenberg, Munich (1959)

Vogel, Ch.: Haftpflichtansprüche aus der zahnärztlichen Chirurgie. *Dtsch. Z. Mund-Kiefer-Gesichtschir.* 3, 3 (1979)

Wagner, W.: *Erregerspektrum und Resistenzsituation bei pyogenen Infektionen im Kiefer- und Gesichtsbereich.* Inaug. Diss., Mainz (1976)

Walter, A. M. and L. Heilmeyer: *Antibiotika-Fibel.* Thieme, Stuttgart (1975)

Wannenmacher, E.: Die Entfernung der dritten Molaren im Unterkiefer. *Dtsch. Zahnärztebl.* 7, 363 (1953)

Ward, T. G.: The split bone technique for removal of lower third molars. *Brit. dent. J.* 101, 297 (1956)

Wassmund, M.: *Lehrbuch der praktischen Chirurgie des Mundes und der Kiefer.* Vol. 1. Meusser, Leipzig (1935)

Welch, J. T. and R. W. Graves: Klassifizierung, Diagnostik und Lokalisierung impaktierter Zähne. In: Slaughter, T. W. and L. J. Boucher, *Impaktierte Zähne, okklusale Artikulation.* Medica, Stuttgart (1980)

Zimmermann, D. C.: Präoperative, chirurgische und postoperative Aspekte der Entfernung impaktierter. In: Slaughter, T. W. and L. J. Boucher, *Impaktierte Zähne, okklusale Artikulation.* Medica, Stuttgart (1980)

Index

Index

(Italicised numbers refer to figures)